M000218556

SECRETS Beyond Aromatherapy

CHAKRA HEALING SECRETS and
ETHERIC COLOUR CODES

Behind the Invisible Etheric Codes of Essential Oils
Chakra & Energy Healing Secrets for the New Era

MYRA SRI

www.myrasri.com

Energy Healing Secrets Series

COPYRIGHT and LEGAL NOTICE

First Published as electronic book in Australia 2012
Revised Edition: 2015
Published by Healing Knowhow™ Publishing,
Suite 2/36 Wallarah Rd,Gorokan, 2263 Australia
*First Printing: **Sept 2015***

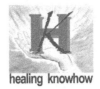

healing knowhow

National Library of Australia Cataloguing-in-Publication entry
Sri, Myra, author
Secrets beyond aromatherapy: chakra healing secrets and etheric colour codes / Myra Sri
ISBN: 9780992392406 (paperback)
Energy healing secrets series ; 1
Includes bibliographical references
Aromatherapy
615.3219

Thank you to my clients, students and colleagues for your encouragement to write this book. And to publish it to other interested light seekers and light bringers.

Blessed be the gifts of Nature, the gifts of Light and the gifts of Gaia. And Blessings to all those who seek more of the Light.

<><><>

CONTENTS

INTRODUCTION

The beauty and power of Essential Oils has been known to us for thousands of years, from Ancient Indian healers to current day Aromatherapists.

Most of us are aware of the use of Essential Oils for a variety of treatments, and most of us have used them for many of those same applications. We are aware of the benefit of using them in massage, in skin care, in emotional re-balancing, in lifting or changing a mood in a room or space and in some cases in treating more serious issues relating to illness or disease.

Our understanding has been generally limited to these everyday and aromatherapy uses.

There are some circles where we are also aware of their use in assisting the nervous system via the brain, to improve and enhance neural function, activity and integration.

There are a number of people who are aware of the advantages of the use of Essential Oils because of the unseen energy vibrations of the oils.

Very few know of their use in this way to treat or enhance the Chakras, meridians, or even the DNA of the Being. Or that Essential Oils can be used in a conscious way and in direct focused application for balancing the energy systems of the body and related chakra energy centers.

Very few are aware of the Colour Codes of Essential Oils.

Very few are aware of their Etheric Language and Activity.

In this book we will explore the language and actions of these Colour Codes and Etheric applications.

We are moving through time and space in an unprecedented way. Some of the proven ways that worked before still work as well, however, they may need an upgrade.

Since 2001 there have been many revelations regarding these upgrades in how we use and process energy. With the various indications by the turnover of the clock of tick-tock time into the new millennium and with the predictions according to the Mayan Long Count Calendar, many things have changed in the perceptions of countless consciousnesses around the globe. New technology has brought us a plethora of information. Some good, some bad.

However, along with this information and the access to information, we have been given the opportunity to discern, to sift through and to learn.

Our beliefs have been challenged, our habitual ways of doing things has been challenged, more of the dark doings of those with dark hearts have been revealed, but also more of those bright lights that shine in the dark have projected further clarity to encourage change and to seize the positive for these current times.

Along with this backdrop, new therapies have emerged, based on some of the old ways. These too are being upgraded as not only new information arises, but the energies that bring these shifts also make changes even in some cases at the cellular level.

We have been dealing with shifts in so many areas, and just as within many our latent codes and memories are resurfacing with the energetic actions of the shifts both on the Planet and off it, so too are the natural and original inhabitants of this globe – that of Earth's plentiful plant life - are also being re-activated.

The original codes of Essential Oils; coming from the plants, their photosynthesis abilities, their anchoring through the trunk, their gifts of love and labor with their fruits and harvest, and the variety of their varied natural substances; all were here to help us. And help us they did. But things have changed and are still changing on this planet.

Because of these shifts and changes, or more accurately alongside them, Essential Oils have taken on a new role, an enhanced ability. Their etheric nature appears to have shifted, to have evolved. The hidden secrets of their invisible colours and their impacts are now being made known and their enhanced functions are aiding in the balancing of our new etheric and subtle body anatomy to meet the demands of these times.

This book endeavours to give a greater awareness not only of the Etheric actions of Essential Oils, but of the cycle and order of Etheric Colours emitted from these amazing gifts of Nature.

Right now they have surely 'come of age'!

Since the turn of this century and the discovery of the new evolved Chakras, the new Chakra anatomy systems have been revealing themselves; some new chakras are now more readily visible or accessible and some are fully evolved. Some of these Chakras were also relating in new ways with aspects of the existing Major Chakras and Higher Chakras, and so were becoming more cohesive and taking on their own organizational identities as new semi-complete systems.

These became individual groups of Chakras that function effectively within themselves for set higher functions.

Now is the perfect time to acquaint one's self with the new evolved ways of these faithful nature oils and of how they are further able to assist us on our own journey and evolution.

This book combines original information and also practical, hands-on applications of the oils for removing energy blocks and bringing comfort to the being. This includes the main energy centers involved as well as which light body and relevant meridians are enhanced and supported by the valuable properties of the oils.

Even the best and most effective of energy workers, LightBringers, and practitioners will find something in here that will enhance their work – whether it is knowledge of the benefits, wisdoms, tips and valuable application techniques or simply knowing which Chakras will benefit the most.

New information and references to the New Chakra Systems that are evolving and operating in these times in tandem with the Major Chakra systems will further enhance any workers effectiveness to deal with the myriad of new symptoms resulting from the conversions of our energy systems to the new and higher New Energy Wave frequencies. To this end there is a limited Glossary included at the end of the book.

It is hoped that the meta-physical applications contained in this book may assist and possibly revolutionize healing work for some, and many LightBringers will experience a new depth to their work with their new found knowledge of the etheric vibrations and actions of Essential Oils.

The Author has attempted to outline the common effects of the etheric aspects and colour vibrations on the energy elements of the Human Energy being – this includes Chakras, meridians and subtle auric or energy fields or bodies. Reference to their emotional, mental, spiritual and in some cases, past life applications and connections have been included.

Any illustrations are the Author's own attempt to convey the energy action of the oil. It is intended that the references found in this book will promote a more enhanced healing experience, a deeper understanding of the issues related, and a greater appreciation of these precious oils and their wonderful gifts right here, right now.

It is with pleasure that the Author shares this knowledge with the public.

Myra Sri

EVOLUTION

The intelligence of the energy Being never failed to amaze me as the new Chakras revealed themselves. As we house more light and uptake more individual responsibility (and inner authority), we have evolved remarkable new subtle body anatomy.

Along with this evolutionary awareness, a new knowing has arrived for many of us, and so my previous use of essential oils simply had to change. Even though they had been a part of my practice from the start, I had also been through a time where I did not require them as before for several years.

But then with the advent of the new era energy shifts and waves, something happened, something seemed to re-awake in them and it suddenly felt as if they had somehow become more alive – their vibrancy was being felt more and more, and it seemed as though they were pleading to work with me again in a different and more conscious way. It was like a hand tapping me on the shoulder and saying 'Pay more attention!' as I began to use them again...

For over 20 years, Vibrational Healing tools and essences had been a natural part of my healing work. Now there was a fresh 'life' about them. And as I worked with the new energy systems, the oils wanted to assist aspects of my work in new ways.

Discovering their etheric colours was a breakthrough for my new and conscious use of them. Discovering the meanings of these colours and new applications was a further revelation.

As I began to work afresh with them, my earlier understandings of their energetic therapeutic applications seemed to be fresh and new and it was as if they were now upgraded with new understandings and capabilities. I found that I was more than appreciative for their amazing gifts and the speedy healings achieved on so many other levels with what I now realized were their enhanced Etheric Properties and Actions of these amazing Colour Codes of Essential Oils.

Along with my knowledge that each Chakra does not simply resonate to one colour alone, I now had the oils with a renewed coding system and a refreshed vigor to bathe the Chakras with the correct codes of colour and energy when and where needed.

Loving colour as I do, and having attempted to yield the artist's brush in creative moments, I was more than delighted to learn of these bountiful etheric colour codes contained in our everyday essential oils. Sharing this accumulation of etheric and practical knowledge with clients and students has further created the demand for a book as a 'proper' documented reference.

Along with the discoveries of the evolving new Chakra systems, I had noted that the basic etheric body colours of the human energy systems also appeared to be changing. Even the Main Chakras were responding differently to colour and vibration. I realized that no longer do most of us reflect (and often poorly at that) the basic opaque paint-box-type colours previously associated with the seven basic colours of the rainbow – some of us are now able to reflect more glorious and colourful hues and iridescences from and through the auric layers and chakras when balanced correctly.

Living in cities can prevent some of these new hues and their tints from shining within and without, as the electromagnetic smog and pollution can lower the frequencies to a paler and poorer version.

In these times it is becoming more important to reconnect back to nature, the land or the sea, purer energies, higher vibrations and natural remedies whenever and wherever possible to sustain us.

It is my firm understanding that the humble oil along with knowledge of its inherent colour codes and abilities will further enhance everyone's experience of the nature and the knowing that is held within each loving oil and hidden within the etheric world itself, and will further enhance and amplify all of your current benefits when used with the increased awareness.

Because of the new dimensions to their etheric energies and uses, this book came into being. I have been truly honored to be part of the evolving energy applications and therapies.

Myra Sri

WHAT ARE THE ETHERIC COLOUR CODES?

We are already aware of the 'smell' or perfume of Essential Oils. We are aware that they may help make us 'feel better'. (And there may be some we may not be able to abide.)

We may also be aware that they are often used in good quality perfumes, and may be added to certain cosmetics or skin care products promoting the use 'natural' ingredients.

However they also possess a hidden life, a powerful aspect, that is not visible to the naked or untrained eye and that cannot normally be seen by the average person.

Each Essential Oil is unique, and just as it has its own individual perfume or fragrance, it has its own coding in the form or vibrational frequency and colour. This is all part of the etheric properties of the oil.

Etheric components of essential oils are due to their composition of volatile oils, which tend to evaporate, becoming ether or etheric. Ether is a primary matter of life and taken in by the nose and skin. It accesses an important part of human consciousness. The unseen energies of oils are the etheric component, they are etheric ('of ether') and so are able to impact and act on the etheric bodies (light bodies and subtle energy bodies).

When we look at colours in a scientific way, we can see that they are part of the visible spectrum of light. When split by a prism, light is made up of all of the colours of the rainbow: Red through to Violet. Each colour has its own frequency or vibration. The frequency aspect of colour is measurable, and yet they occupy only an extremely limited spectrum on the frequencies scale; with many frequencies not at all visible to the naked eye, such as the infra-red rays and ultra-Violet rays.

Other frequencies that do not allow themselves to be seen as visible colour may register as sound, sonic electronic or radio wave frequencies. There are many vibrational frequencies that make up our world that are entirely invisible to our eye, but are nevertheless very real and important. [Interestingly, we are now accustomed to text messaging, e-mail and a whole variety of electronic and frequency broadcasts that pass through the atmosphere daily, and every millisecond... yet we can see none of these, even when the messages include coloured photographs or pictures!]

Our main colour spectrum usually goes from Red, which is the longest energy wave with the slowest vibration, through the colours of Orange, Yellow, Green then Blue and Indigo to Violet, which is the fastest frequency with the shortest wave. The rainbow is a faithful representation of the order of the colours

Generally we are able to see these rainbow colours. But we cannot see their frequency, though we can register their impact on us... such as when a colour annoys us or makes us feel calm or tends to make us feel excited. We may even have an adverse reaction to a colour that we dislike intensely or that tends to make us feel sick or just plain 'blah'. This may be because it is triggering something in us, or that has affected us from our past. A competent Kinesiologist can assist us to balance to a particular colour frequency, which can also clear the associated negative reaction.

COLOUR FREQUENCIES – COLOUR CODES

Each colour has an etheric frequency, an unseen colour frequency that impacts upon our energetic frequency body in a particular way.

These unseen colour vibrations create specific actions on the Etheric body, which is the underpinning or the scaffolding if you like of the physical matter, and the matrix for the energy bodies.

We have vitality, life-force, electrical and magnetic living energy in the body that can be monitored and measured in frequencies, and even photographed or tracked with electronic devices. When we take a look at this energetic subtle body anatomy, we become aware of the etheric makeup of the physical and unseen energy bodies that everyone possesses.

Even religion can attest to the 'auras' or halos of the saints or sainted ones. Kirlian photography developed by the Russians has proven the aura of plants and people for decades now.

These energy 'halos' are invisible to the naked eye unless one has specific frequency reading devices or spectacles, or one has clairvoyant-psychic or aura-reading abilities.

We each of us have our own electrical field, and this responds to frequencies, and to colour.

So too, plants possess their own particular colour range and frequencies of energy that translates into specific and individual colour codes and 'recipes'. These etheric colours, these colour codes, exist for every Essential Oil. And in the action of the colour, in the specific progression of the individual colour frequencies within each Essential Oil lay the secret and the key to the code.

Most oils have not just one colour, but many. And may even have a simultaneous combining action at the same time! This can literally bathe the etheric and energetic parts of the body with a delightful kaleidoscope of delicious soothing, nurturing or healing frequencies.

It is this progression of colour and their inherent code that creates the changes, and knowledge of these enhances our conscious use of them for the most beneficial results.

<><><>

ONE INTERESTING COLOUR EXPERIMENT

There was a TV program some time ago about a **men's prison in Houston, Texas,** that painted all of its walls a particular colour. They also proceeded to put all of the inmates in the same colour spectrum, including socks and shoes. It was reported that return prisoners dropped off, that there were no repeat offenders, and that there was no trouble in the prison whilst these colours were in operation!

The colour they used was Pink!

Some commentators thought it was because the men felt humiliated in Pink, a 'girl's' colour, and some of the inmates thought the same too. But Pink is renowned for its ability to bring acceptance, and even self-love into play. It is a heart colour, actually one of the 'new' colours of the Chakra system!

(This experiment was first trialed in San Jose, California, at the Santa Clara County Jail – then refined and applied in Houston, Texas.)

<><><>

Oil Colour Codes and the New Energy Wave

Ancient knowledge has been reviving and re-emerging over the last 30 years or so and continues to do so. As the new frequencies bring to our consciousness those parts of us that have been forgotten, dis-connected or negated we can use oils in a more conscious and mindful way to re-activate and heal so as to enhance our journey and ease our path.

Certain ancient subtle body anatomy that was dormant (though often present), is now re-awakening. We are also developing *New* subtle body anatomy - which has been evolving, and is now ready for alignment and activation.

It is now time to anchor the new incoming energies appropriately and in a new way in these current times.

Because of these changes, it is my opinion, observation and experience that the effect, power and action of Essential Oils is changing. We are expanding in our innate understanding and use of them. Not only that, their use in self help healing is becoming not only more popular, but more comprehensive and accessible.

It is so easy to enhance your energy fields, energy, sense of well-being and your aura with the simple healing technique of working with Essential Oils through directed breathing in a conscious and etheric way.

We are being challenged to ensure that we are anchored as never before as we continue to further venture through time and space, and Essential Oils have taken on a new mission, and a new way of assisting. As we have evolved, so the gifts of these precious and powerful oils have certainly moved up a notch to assist us with our evolution.

The planet herself testifies to the changes in consciousness. Freedom of communication and information is making available to millions what was hard to access, or difficult to share. Our understanding of connection has taken on a global perspective, and this is moving into a galactic perspective.

Just as our technology has advanced, so too have we energetically advanced, and in the same way as we are attempting to keep up with the leaps of technological advances and the development of more complicated electronic applications and devices, so too we are learning to 'drive' our new energetic anatomy.

As the Planet shifts on her axis, and moves slightly differently through space we move into different wavebands and frequencies. Some of this is quite new for humanity in relatively recent evolutionary experience. And we are relating to nature and our position in space-time slightly differently.

As we register these new frequencies and attempt to align to them, Essential oils that are used correctly can speed up the alignment process and 'key' us in to the shifts and changes with more ease.

THE NEW ENERGY WAVES

VIBRATIONAL and ENERGETIC HEALING in THE NEW ENERGY WAVE

WHAT IS 'THE NEW ENERGY WAVE'

What do we *mean* by the term 'New Energy Wave'?

We are all aware of the force of gravity on our planet. We are aware of the power of solar flares to affect all our electrical equipment. Some of you are also aware of what can happen in delays or in creating communication problems when the planet Mercury goes retrograde approximately once every three months for about three weeks.

Well, right now the planet is moving through some interesting frequencies in space. There are a lot of planetary alignments that have not occurred for over 26,000 years, and as these planets move into alignment, they affect and so shift and change the normal movements of space winds, and the way of the electromagnetic relationships of the set paths of the planets.

This impacts on our world.

We are also experiencing shifts within our planet, such as global climate changes, increased weather pattern changes, increased earthquakes, tsunamis, and other natural phenomenon.

In short, we are experiencing changes both above, from outer space, and below, from the planet we stand upon.

And many of us are seeking new ways of riding these new waves.

As we move in space through and past the end-time of the *Kali Yuga* – which was indicated by and coincided with the Mayan Long Count Calendar which ended in December 2012 - and align with the *Galactic Center-Galactic Anticenter* axis - Sacred Sites across the globe further indicated these cosmological positions, when they pointed to Sagittarius and Gemini in December 2012 - we experience new vibrations.

These vibrations meet with our energy fields, and where there is resistance, they 'shake' up and attempt to integrate. When they cannot penetrate and flow through easily, we experience a variety of 'symptoms' or discomforts.

Many of us are evolving, and as we evolve, we reveal the new subtle body anatomy and specialized Chakra Systems that are enhancements to our current Major Chakra anatomy. This has been progressing for some time, as we move into the new and higher frequencies.

There is talk of 'Ascension', which may be helpful to think of as 'Upgrades' of our systems, frequencies and purpose, as well as our destination.

This creates changes.

This creates growth.

With growth there is sometimes pain as we leave an old garment behind to don a new and better one. This is the process that many of us are in right now.

<><><>

We are 'converting' - 'upgrading'... - and maybe in some way we are quite possibly 'ascending'... or at least being given the opportunity to do so...

The myriad of new symptoms resulting from these conversions of our energy systems to the new and higher 'New Energy Wave' frequencies do not all lend themselves to resolution through some of the old methods and techniques.

3 Dimensional techniques help 3D issues, but we are moving into 4D and 5D frequencies – and in some cases some of you are already moving into other dimensions.

Maintaining balance within will assist us, as we are being forced to discover new arts of inner healing as we encounter and deal with the many changes surrounding us right now.

A New Role — Vibrational Energy Healing

Essential Oils are an amazing form of concentrated and focused planetary and cosmic energy in the embodiments of plants, flowers, lipids and other natural substances. Their application and relationship to us and to the living (the 'living' includes all life forms, whether human or animal, no matter where they sit on the consciousness or evolutionary scale) is shifting and thus coming into a different association with humanity, and the individual human energy systems in particular.

Not only can we enjoy their application on a sensual and conscious aromatherapy level, we can now use them as a very real healing tool that, when combined with intent and consciousness, takes a quantum energy leap and works on a vibrational energy healing level.

We are already aware of the effects of Essential Oils on the Nervous System and the Brain, studies supporting what the ancient wise knew well.

With the advent of energy measuring, energy monitoring and energy photography, we can also verify what psychics and clairvoyants have seen or known for centuries: Essential oils have etheric colours and properties.

ETHERIC PROPERTIES OF ESSENTIAL OILS

Invisible etheric energies unseen by the ordinary human eye pervade and saturate essential oils.

Because of the innate refinement of their Vibrational frequency energy, their qualities are able to infiltrate and pass through human Etheric fields, creating vibrational healing changes as they go when applied correctly. Topical (on the surface of the skin) application is not the only method of using oils.

I will attempt to demonstrate this to you with everyday ideas – and please forgive any mixed metaphors.

Such as if you can imagine what happens with say smoke from a fire, or a cigarette, and how it passes through into hair and clothing, you may possibly begin to imagine the emanations of the vibrations from essential oils.

Or imagine someone having eaten heaps of garlic, and you can literally smell it oozing out of their skin.

[At a deeper level, imagine x-rays passing through even dense bone. The energies of essential oils can pass through into the energetic structure when used correctly, and also because of their very nature as they are in harmony with humanity.]

However, their action is even stronger than this, as the fineness of their frequencies can penetrate more than smoke can.

They can be absorbed and pass through cellular barriers. This is seen clearly when applying Lavender to the wrist or temple points. The Lavender is absorbed directly into the blood stream, usually safely as it has so many soothing applications, and as you probably are already aware, it also reaches the nervous system and the brain. This helps to calm, relax and soothe.

Oils generally will not penetrate where they are not welcome, as they are generally not aligned to force or infringement toward others.

Continual use of the same oil day after day over a period of time may be okay except in certain circumstance. Most oils are safe to use often, however some need a rest – for instance, only use Juniper Oil judiciously, and cease for a rest after using for 3 months as the strength of their detoxification abilities will build up in the system. So go easy with this oil. Though occasional use will speed up release of toxins in both the physical and the energy bodies.

[If you suspect you are pregnant, please take care with essential oils and check for their safety in use!]

<><><>

ESSENTIAL OILS AND VIBRATIONAL FREQUENCY

We are becoming more and more aware that everything in the universe vibrates at its own particular frequency. Living creatures, plants, objects - everything has a frequency, even disease. Kirlian photography went a long way toward proving invisible energy emanations from plant life. This has evolved to the ability to take common 'Aura' photos with specially designed cameras which register more than just the colour light waves that are visible to the naked eye.

In 1992 the first frequency monitor in the world was built by Bruce Tainio of Tainio Technology, an independent division of Eastern State University in Cheny, Washington. The Tainio monitor determined that the average frequency of the healthy human body during normal daytime is in the range of 62 to 72 Hz. It also showed that when the frequency drops, this jeopardizes the immune system. If the frequency rate drops to 58 Hz, then usually cold and flu symptoms begin to appear. At 55 Hz diseases like Candida can be triggered, and at 52 Hz this can register as Epstein Bar. Cancer is usually vibrating at 42 Hz and below.

This study of frequencies can raise important questions regarding the frequency of substances we ingest or absorb regularly. Many pollutants can lower our body's vibrational frequency. Processed or canned foods usually have a frequency of zero. Fresh produce has up to 15 Hz and 25 Hz for organic produce, dried herbs from 12 to 22 Hz, and fresh herbs can register from 20 to 27 Hz.

Essential oils start at a frequency of 52 Hz and can go up as high as 320 Hz, as in the Turkish Rose Oil.

Clinical research shows that essential oils have the highest frequency of any natural substance known to man. They can create a condition where bacteria, virus, fungus and disease simply cannot survive. On the physical level, this gives us a tool for self help on a practical and often affordable level. On an etheric or energetic level, they can act in a metaphysical way to clear out energetic viruses, remove energetic contaminations and amplify energy work.

ORIGINS OF ESSENTIAL OILS

The use of essential oils is recorded as far back as 5000 years.

Ancient Ayurvedic texts make reference to their powerful properties for healing the body and the mind. Ayurveda is part of the ancient Traditional Indian Vedic systems of healing and nurturing.

The ancient Egyptians had many uses for essential oils, extracting them by infusion. Common uses were cosmetics, healing, food preservation and even embalming. They were also used for religious ceremonies and making incense. Every god or goddess in ancient Egypt had their own particular essence. Cleopatra is said to have bathed in rose petals. (Whether added to a milk bath or a water bath, most of us will have heard about this luxurious and extravagant beauty treatment.)

The ancient Chinese also used essential oils for religious purposes and for healing, massage, and incense making. Incense burning was and is an important part of their religious ceremonies.

In India, some of the temples were built out of sandalwood in an attempt to join the gods and their worshipers in fragrant unity.

The ancient Greeks, who owe much of their knowledge to the Egyptians, also linked essences to the spirit. The Greeks considered scents a direct gift from the gods. They believed that the afterworld, or paradise they called Elysium, was a place where perfumed rivers flow.

However, it appears that it was the Romans who were mainly responsible for the spread and popularity of essential oils in Europe, who used them for their fragrances, healing and cosmetic properties.

HOW DO THEY WORK?

Essential Oils are amazingly effective because they can reach the blood stream in 20 minutes to half an hour maximum through their speedy ability to be absorbed through the skin when used topically. After testing for safety in the oils neat form, when it is applied neat as with Lavender, absorption takes only minutes. (Where possible, pre-test the oil on a small patch of skin.)

Their fragrance also activates nerve cells in the nasal cavity sending impulses to the limbic system, an area of the brain associated with emotions and memory. The Olfactory centres in the nasal area has direct access to the brain and its memory and emotion centres.

Most essential oils are antiseptic and some are antibacterial. It has also been shown that a few drops of essential oil before your daily skin routine may actually double or even triple your skin care benefits.

DO THEY AFFECT EVERYONE THE SAME WAY?

Each essential oil has a well-know biological effect but since it also affects the central nervous system, each person reacts according to his or her condition.

Used normally, the same essential oil can have a relaxing or tonifying effect depending on the body's requirement. A good example is Lavender oil. In eighty percent of cases it is soothing, but has a contrary tonifying effect on some people though this may depend upon what is occurring within their bodies and energy fields at the time.

In the same way each etheric colour will have the appropriate affect for that particular individual.

With the new frequencies and the development new subtle body anatomies, these frequencies are of immense benefit. Will they affect you all in the same way? No!

...As your anatomy will distinctly reflect exactly where you are at in your personal transformation and purpose process, so each individual will show different aspects of growth and thus the need will differ person to person. But the effect of the oil will not differ.

<><><>

WHICH OIL IS RIGHT FOR ME?

Generally the oil that attracts you most is the one that works best for you.

Deciding which oil to use is generally an individual decision, and often an intuitive one. It can also be based on its perfume, how one feels at the time, and what one knows about the oil itself.

Knowing about their energetic and healing properties is therefore extremely useful, and can often demonstrate just why one has chosen a particular oil.

For even more revealing application, **simple Self Test Kinesiology** will prove extremely helpful in discovering the best oil for the job at the present moment that it is needed.

A word: Do not choose an oil because of its etheric colour alone whilst trying to match it to a Chakra.

Chakras can become over-energized, and applying more of the same colour will not necessarily help, and may hinder. Even the Base Chakra, known for its Red (Pink in an evolved being) on occasion may need its opposite of Green to settle and soothe it.

ARE THEY SAFE? WHAT ABOUT SIDE EFFECTS?

Baths and Point Massage

The body generally tolerates essential oils well. It's important not to use pure oils directly onto the skin or in the bath water as they can irritate the skin.

Depending on your intended use, they can be diluted in your shower gel, bath product or vegetable oils like sweet almond oil, Jojoba oil or avocado oil, or in a cream or moisturizer base. You can even buy a neutral base cream especially to dilute your essential oils.

Some oils may cause temporary skin reactions if used neat or undiluted - amongst these are Thyme, Oregano, Cinnamon, Peppermint and Lemongrass oils and possibly others. These work better in a base carrier oil such as Sweet Almond Oil or even Olive Oil. Nut oils can work well with essential oils for the purpose of skin nourishment.

Other essential oils may make your skin more sensitive to the sun and are best not be used for twelve hours before sun exposure. These are Bergamot essences as well as Lemon, Grapefruit and Mandarin essences. Others must be used with due care, and notice taken of any precautions recommended.

USING THE POWER OF ESSENTIAL OILS

HOW DO I USE THEM?

There are many ways to use essential oils. As I have mentioned, their applications have been revived and they are now available to use on a different level and dimension, as we move through the New Energy Wave.

Essential Oils can be used by inhaling direct from its bottle. They can also be diluted in carrier vegetable oils that support and diffuse them, making their perfume and effect less concentrated for topical application. They can be added as drops direct into bath water or for hydrating the skin when cleansing.

For energy work, for self help healing, and for therapists facilitating others in session work, the following section contains some powerful yet simple techniques that are highly recommended.

This section indicates some useful and proven techniques for the applications of oils in a healing situation. Please also use any other safe technique you feel comfortable with.

ENERGY WORK APPLICATION SUGGESTIONS

It is wise to always replace the lid immediately or as soon as possible after use, to protect the potency, life and strength of the essential oil. The exception would be if you momentarily use the lid to inhale.

Always replacing the lid when not directly using maintains its etheric strength and quality, and serves to prevent any loss of etheric vitality or effectiveness.

Most of the following techniques can be used during an Energy Healing session or with most therapies. The **Meditation or Journaling** technique is a great way to get in depth with an issue, and to reach understandings, if you really want to dig under an issue or block that you are holding.

If you create your own blend or mix of oils, always test on the skin for reaction. A good suggestion is to only ever use blue or brown glass bottles for safe and protective storage. If you are using the oil within a couple of days or so, you might get away with some other form of container, but glass is best and coloured glass even better.

Conscious Breathing Technique:

Focusing on the oil and its etheric colours can enhance, amplify or quicken the action of the oil. You can use the lid to the bottle, or the bottle itself as long as you don't tilt it too much and spill in onto the face – these are powerful substances, and some can aggravate the skin if not diluted. You can dab a couple of drops onto a tissue and use this to breathe in the etheric vibrations, waving it gently under the nose without touching it, so as to ensure it enters both nostrils, and to gain access to both sides of the brain as you inhale.

Always be aware that breathing inward assists with drawing the energies within your body and energy fields, and breathing out is just as important, as the outward breath carries what is being loosened, resolved, liberated or no longer required. The colours create change, and just as the oils used the channel of breath to enter, so does the origin of the imbalance need a channel of escape.

Conscious Directed Inhaling Technique:

When you work with consciously breathing in the etheric colours of the oils, you engage with it at a more powerful level, as your consciousness can enhance the colour effects.

To not only breathe in, but also to *Direct* your breathing into an area that needs healing or attention will greatly enhance the oils action.

For instance, if you are working with a Chakra, you can direct the oil into the particular Chakra location or area, and assist the oil at a deeper level. As your conscious mind recognizes what you are working with, and the oil engages you energetically, you begin to call into alignment other energy bodies that may be out of balance connected with this area.

If you are working with an emotion and feel unsettled within your nervous system or in the stomach, *directing* the oil into these areas whilst drawing it in on the breath will facilitate cellular releases of these buried or absorbed emotions. The inward *Directed* breath takes the colour energies to the area, the outward breath releases the unwanted or discharging energies from your body and energy fields.

Remember, what has gone in must also come out. Energy just doesn't disappear, but it can change and transmute.

Auric Wiping:

Placing a couple of drops on a tissue, you can apply the power of the oil into the light body that needs balance wherever it is required, in the place that requires it – this may possibly be over a particular meridian, or it may be around a particular chakra. It also may need it in a particular light body at a place of congestion (that may not be obviously connected to physical anatomy), to remove gunked up or stagnant energies.

Atmospheric Clearing:

Using simple Sprays assists with clearing a space, or shifting the vibration to a more conducive level and to bring more ease or peace. Oil Burners are popular for background ambience and most can be 'set and forget'. But the spray action seems to be more energetically active in stimulating and clearing quickly.

Sprays can be used during Energy Work at specific stages, to assist in clearing any dense vibration that has resulted through the release of blocked energy. This can assist in clearing the space and the etheric bodies to either calm and center, or to prepare for accessing the next level of energy facilitation. In the best clinics, there are usually at least a couple of sprays for different purposes.

A simple Spray can be made by using a few drops of the appropriate essential oil or mix of oils (know what you are doing before you combine oils) with water and some oil solubiliser drops to allow the oil to be soluble and to mix with the water.

Physical Applications:

Oils in carrier oils such as Almond, Jojoba or Hemp oil can be used for specific actions in Massage, and to apply on Acupuncture Points. Massage allows for absorption directly through the skin into the nervous system and circulation. When applied to points, you are applying the energy directly to the energy blockage on the meridian or lymphatic node. This can assist in stimulating the energy flow again, and in moving stuck physical energy.

Sometimes the body and being needs a couple of different ways of application in order to break through some blockages.

Meridian Work:

You will find a diagram for meridian application at the end of this section. You can massage of apply the diluted oil along the meridian line to ease stress or blocks in that meridian. Always apply in the direction of the meridian flow. I have placed them in order according to the flow of meridian-to-meridian in TCM. Sometimes the block in one meridian is caused by a block in a previous meridian.

Chakra Work:

You will find a diagram for chakra application at the end of this section. These are shown as placed at the front of the body, but most Chakras run directly through the body, so you can access the Chakra via the front or back of the body.

Being mindful of what a Chakra is will give benefit to the work performed with the essential oils, or indeed with any vibrational medicine or application. Giving thought to the Chakra function can also be of added benefit.

The Extra-Ordinary Chakras are not shown in this book. The Extra-Ordinary Chakras include the Higher Chakras, Human Earthing Chakras, Psychic Body Chakras and the Signal Chakra System. The Minor Chakras that relate to organs, joints and glands can be accessed when working on the body, and a basic knowledge of anatomy and physiology can assist with this.

Combination Applications:

There are occasions when you may feel you need several of the above for true efficacy or effectiveness. Not only Directed Breathing is required, but also Auric Wiping, and maybe a spray to finish off.

Word of Warning: When performing combinations like this, don't try to use too many oils in one hit, unless you are already a good healer. (A good healer can hold the space of several frequencies to good effect.) A novice or self helper may find that too much is happening, or a toxic release crisis may get triggered. So to be safe, keep it to only one or two oils at a time. This way you can also observe and monitor the effects, so that you can actively work toward your greater health and well-being in a responsible and practical way.

Kinesiology Diagnosis

An amazing tool for assisting with choosing the right tool, the right oil, the right meridian, the right spot, the right Chakra, right now... is Kinesiology. Simple Self Testing Kinesiology is of amazing value. In the book *'Secrets Behind Energy Fields'* I share the technique that *anyone* can learn; Simple Finger Test kinesiology.

Affirmation Meditation / Journaling:

Working with oils consciously can be a powerful self support and self healing technique.

If there is an affirmation that you particularly want to clear any imbalance on or you want to really embed into your energy bodies, this is a great way to go.

Set aside regular time, without any interruptions, say 15 - 20 minutes. Set it up so that you can be undisturbed, agitated or bothered (go to the toilet, get a cup of tea or glass of water, take the phone off the hook, lock the door, etc).

Write your affirmation, then inhale the oil while you hold the thought you have just written. You can place a few drops on a tissue for ease of use and to maintain preservation of the bottled oil. Allow it to flow through your physical and energy bodies. Pause a moment to see what arises. Listen to what your thoughts have to say, and write whatever you hear in your mind down on the opposite page of your notebook.

Do not focus on what comes up in response. Focus only on what you are writing [planting in your mind] and on allowing the oil to do its work in your energy systems and body.

Refocus on the statement or affirmation you desire to become part of your reality, and keep repeating as above. Continue for several days (usually 7 – 10 days) and note daily your reactions and awareness's.

If you stop before you have finished your intended days or affirmation numbers (you can use a timer, diary, calendar or any other tracking system to be sure), you MUST start again. If you miss a day, you MUST start all over again from day 1 – whatever number of days you have committed to, you MUST see it through to uninterrupted completion for this to take a real hold in your energy systems and neurology. It is well worth the effort, though.

This is a clearing process, and not an analyzing process, though this technique can be adapted for either.

When you have completed this, you can launch into another statement you wish to 'plant' within yourself, though it is wise to initially give yourself a few days rest if you are new to this. This allows for integration and for the next 'layer' to emerge.

Myra Sri

MAJOR CHAKRA POSITIONS

Illustrated below are the positions of the commonly recognized Main Chakra System.

Each Chakra has an associated colour which ranges from red for the Base Chakra through to Violet for the Crown Chakra. Colour Plate can be downloaded at: http://www.myrasri.com/chart-for-book-buyers

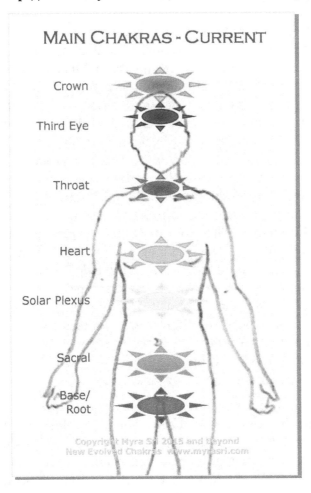

THE MAIN CHAKRAS

Some of you may well already know about the Chakras and simply require the individual oils information to enhance your working knowledge and healing effectiveness. However, for those who are not fully conversant with them, included here are some of the common and major attributes or functions of the Main Chakras.

The purpose of the Chakras, which are wheels of energy often seen as light and colour frequencies, is to step down cosmic and incoming energies so as to be usable at a correct frequency to maintain harmonic resonance in the body, depending on its frequency and associated colour vibration or frequency. The Chakras also feed the etheric body, which in turn feeds the physical body in order to assist with regeneration. The use of the correct and appropriate related or supportive colour will assist in blending incoming frequencies with the individual Chakra colour. This helps the Chakra to process and maintain its function in integrity. The related colour is that which carries its original frequency, such as red for the Base and green for the Heart, as listed below. However, there are occasions when the Chakra is over-energised and it requires a complementary (opposite) colour or an allied colour (similar but with another colour to calibrate the frequency slightly differently) in order to reset or balance down its over-energy as opposed to over-charging in order to boost an under-energised Chakra up.

All Chakras operate independently of each other, yet they can also provide feedback to each other. Sometimes a Chakra may affect its neighbour, but not necessarily so. There are also resonant links between them, as the Base can be balanced by resonating it with the Crown Chakra, the Sacral Chakra can be balanced by resonating it with the Third Eye Chakra, and Solar Plexus with the Throat, whilst the Heart is sometimes used to bring all Chakras into balance.

The Chakras are generally in a cone type shape, with a narrower end that originates in the body closely aligned to nervous system groups and centres, the Chakra increasing in diameter as it emerges from the physical body to be visible outside of the body to those with psychic or energetic perception vision or abilities, as well as energy reading devices. They emit and receive energy vibrations and frequencies in their widening circles of energetic 'radar', and the energetic make-up constitutes of both a clockwise and a counter-clockwise circular spiral motions. Through the centre of the body there tends to be a central channel of energy that links each of the Chakras together, creating a line of energy from body base to the crown and back.

Much has been written about these Chakras and in comparisons of some models, there may appear to be some overlapping of functionality. The truth is to be found in being able to ascertain either the correct attribute or function, or the correct model to work with for a particular body type, or soul type.

Finding the actual functionality of your client's or your own Chakra is the key to discovering if there is any dys-function-ality that requires addressing.

Let the following be a guide only.

BASE CHAKRA

This Chakra associated with the colour Red and its function is connected with Life force and energy, life and death, survival issues, and physical foundations in life. This Chakra is located near the base of the spine, hence its name; it helps us to ground, and is related to action. This is the in-body Chakra that helps to connect us to the evolved out-of-body Chakras below the Earth's surface (the new Earthing Chakras).

SACRAL CHAKRA

Associated with the colour Orange, and located in the pelvic area, this is a feeling Chakra and mainly concerned with emotion, family, nurturing and comforts. It is related to emotional foundations, feeling, sexuality and connectedness with others.

SOLAR PLEXUS CHAKRA

The colour Yellow is the theme with this Chakra which is located near the stomach region, and it is primarily focused on one's will and desires. Yearnings, assimilation of ideas, control issues, how we connect with others, mental foundations and intuition are keywords.

HEART CHAKRA

Placed in the heart region, the heart Chakra is related to love; of self and others as well as acceptance of life. Its usual colour is Green, though in certain instances it prefers Pink. This choice can be based on a Soul preference or purpose for being. This Chakra seeks to balance will, love and expression harmoniously.

THROAT CHAKRA

Associated with the colour Blue and located in the neck and throat region, this Chakra is concerned with truth – giving and speaking our own truth. It is also related to self-expression, communication, and the exchange and balance of the giving and receiving energies.

THIRD EYE CHAKRA

Located on the forehead, it is associated with inner and outer sight and resonates to the colour of Indigo. Imagination, imaging our future, seeing possibilities, seeing the bigger picture, clarity in thinking and finding solutions are all connected with this Chakra.

CROWN OR CORONAL CHAKRA

Associated with the colour of Purple or Violet, this Chakra is generally acknowledged as the spiritual Chakra. Located at the top of the head, it can also connect one with the Higher or Upper Chakras that sit above the head and out-of-the-body.

The next level of tier of Chakras upwards, are the Higher Chakras, which sit in a different etheric level, though they communicate with the Main Chakras.

MAIN MERIDIANS – START & END POINTS

Start position and end point of the meridians, together with yin / yang energy identification.

Oils (in carrier oil) may be applied at the beginning and end of meridian, or along the meridian line. They can also be used at various points along the meridian – preferably some knowledge is required for this. The yin / yang notation indicates the usual energy flow of the meridian.

1. **STOMACH & SPLEEN**
   a. STOMACH Under Eye to Second Toe   yang
   b. SPLEEN Outside Big Toe to Under Arm   yin
   c. HEART In Armpit to Inside Little Finger   yin

2. **SMALL INTESTINE & BLADDER**
   a. SMALL INTESTINE Outer Little Finger Nail to Ear   yang
   b. BLADDER Mid Eyebrow to Outer Little Toe   yang

3. **CIRCULATION-SEX & KIDNEY**
   a. KIDNEY Bottom of Foot to Collar Bone   yin
   b. CIRC-SEX Above Nipple to Inside Second Finger   yin

4. **TRIPLE WARMER & GALL BLADDER**
   a. TRIPLE WRMR Outer Third Finger Nail to Eye Edge   yang
   b. GALL BLADDER Outer Eye Edge to Outer Little Toe   yang

5. **LIVER & LUNG**
   a. LIVER Outer Big Toe Nail to Mid Ribcage   yin
   b. LUNG Lung Side to Outer Thumb   yin

6. **LARGE INTESTINE & CENTRAL & GOVERNING**
   a. LARGE INTESTINE First Finger Nail to Side Nose   yang
   b. CENTRAL Pubic Area to Chin   yin
   c. GOVERNING Pubic Area to Under Nose   yang

MERIDIANS ILLUSTRATION

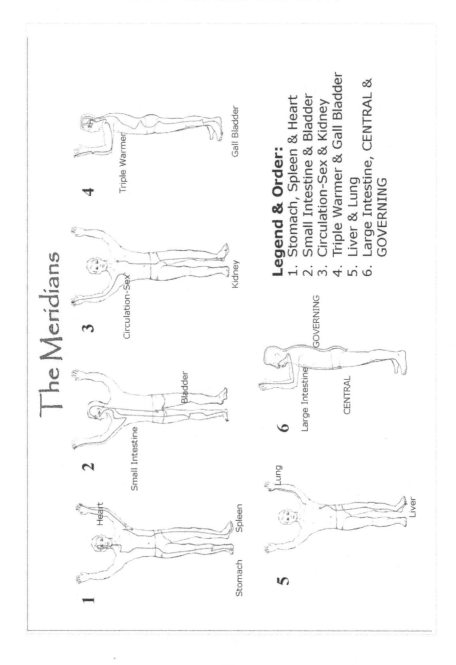

Myra Sri

INDIVIDUAL ESSENTIAL OIL CODES

In this section we will give you the Colour Code and the sequences of these for the Essential Oil, as well as the actions on the energetic and etheric bodies.

The focus will be on the unseen frequencies, rather than on their common recognized uses, though there may be some mention of these as a natural consequence.

Disclaimer:

The benefits cited above and throughout this book are for information only. Please consult a qualified aroma-therapist or holistic health practitioner before using essential oils if you are uncertain.

Please take the 'usual precautions' which are: choose good quality essential oils where possible, test for reactivity if using on the skin, mix with a base or carrier oil for massage and avoid ingesting unless of oral grade. Always check it is safe to use during pregnancy.

It also means checking for the quality of the oil, and if unsure of its possible effects, do a test for reaction: a drop on cotton-wool in the elbow crease for a three minutes or so. If red, a rash or irritation, discontinue or repeat the test in a diluted version on another spot. If still irritation, avoid use.

A usual Dilution for topical use is 15-20 drops in 2 ounces of base oil. *Always check for a reaction.*

INDIVIDUAL OIL COLOUR CODE SUMMARY CHART

Here is a summary, with detailed information following.

OIL	KEYWORDS / ACTION	ETHERIC COLOURS +
BASIL	Self Responsibility, Self-Esteem, Self-Judgment, Self-Limitation, Integrity, Spiritual Joy. Conscious Choices, Renewed Vitality. Manifestation. Brain Activation	Green, Coppery-Turquoise, Peacock Blue, Lavender, Silver-Tin
BENZOIN	Attracts, Soothe & Stimulate, Abundance, Depression	Orange, Red, Deep Amber Gold With Little Blue
BERGAMOT	Opens The Heart, Calms Mental Body, Shock, Bitterness, Depression, Negative Thoughts, Power, Joy & Grace	Deep Greens, Deep Blues to Indigo, Bronze or Copper Feathered Magenta, Orange Spirals
CAJEPUT	Dysfunctional /Abusive Relationships, Male Traits Of Control, Domination Integrates To Receptivity, Fulfill Own Needs, Sexual Issues, Inertia, Self Expression, True Spiritual Love	Orange-InfraRed, Silver, Green Spectrum
CARNATION	Protection, Past Life and Reincarnation Issues, Soul Memories, Life Force, Grounding, Emotional Objectivity, Learning, Focus	Rich Pink-Mauve, Blue, Gold-Silver with Green Flecks
CEDARWOOD	Security & Protection, Clarity, Focus, Direction, Dispel Fantasy Projections, Energy Flow, True Spiritual Love, Hope & Faith For Hearts Desires	Blue-Green Tinged With Deep Orange & Purple
CHAMOMILE	Calms Conscious Mind, Peace, Anger, Loneliness, Nervous System, Abandonment, Grief, Stress, Death Wishes, Lost Love, Heartbreak, Divine Right Timing, Life Transitions, Ghosts	Turquoise, Bluish-Purple, Green, Gold, Silver, White

CINNAMON	Transitions, Past Life Healing, Cellular Memory, Dogma Victim & Enslavement Issues, Power, Abuse. <u>Related Issues:</u> Anger, Abundance, Lack of Happiness, Attachments	Red, Green, Orange, Blue
CITRONELLA	Nervous System, Sugar Imbalances/ Lost Joy, Quick Anger, Comfort & Courage to Resolve Conflicts, Parasitics	Tannish-Orange tinged Red, Yellow
CLARY SAGE	Stops Mind Chatter, Stillness Of Joy, Mental Focus, Confusion, Paranoia, Obsessive Thoughts, Dense Energy Of Depression/ Sorrow, Burdens, Crisis, Anguish/Anxiety, Kidney/Lungs	Deep Blue, Gold, Yellow, Magenta
CLOVE (BUD)	Auric Clearing, Emotional Re-Connection, Root Of Pain, Self Expression, Shock, Joy, Gentle Power, Kundalini, Grounding	Orange, Red, Violet tinged with Teal Green & Gold
FENNEL	Fears Of Lack, Substituting Food Or Other Substances For Love, Weight Issues, Self-Rejection, Thyroid, Self-Nourishment, Past Life Experiences - Famine, Survival or Weight / Power Associations	Yellow/Lemon, Coppery-Green, Light Green, Tiny Red Stars in Clear/Transparent
FRANKINCENSE	Spiritual Purpose, Growth & Choice, Denial, Life Force, Integrity, Mastery, Soul Memories, I Am, Serenity	Silver-Gold Yellow turning into Silvery Mauve/Blue with deep Blue Flame
GARDENIA	Peace, Attract Good Vibrations	Blue, Mauve/Purple, Gold, Pink
GERANIUM	Sense of Safety, Internal Conflicts, Broken Heart, Unite Soul Fragments, Abandonment, Isolation, Shame, Divine Grace, Freedom of Joyous Love	Pink-Green, Gold
GRAPEFRUIT	Calm Mind Chatter, Inner Source Directives, Beliefs & Karmic Imprints, Fragmented Personality, Depression, Auric Density, Thoughtforms, Soul Purpose, New Realities, Core Energy, Mercury Retrograde	Light and Dark Emerald Green, Violet, Yellow, Gold Flakes, Magenta

JASMINE	Good For Auric Holes, Anxiety, Protective, Self-Esteem, Tension, Confidence to Overcome Immediate Problems	Gold, Blue, Pink, Green, Violet, Silver
JUNIPER	Patience, Soul Group Connection, Heart Alignment, Lost Faith, Feeling Love, Stagnant Energies, Pagan Lifetimes, Fairies & Elves	Silver Threads, White-Light, Blue
LAVENDER	Eases Heartache, Reduces Tension and Stress, Enhances Sense of Security, Builds Self Trust, Grace, Allows Relaxation, Soothes Turmoil and Promotes Peace, Aids Sleep, Soothe Nervous System, Allows for New Intuitive Info	Silver-Gold, Blue-Green
LEMON	Inner Joy & Optimism, Throat Chakra, Sharpens Mind, Alcohol Addiction Released From Cellular Memory, Cleansing, Cynicism, Scattered, Detox	Green, Yellow/Goldish, Slightly Violet
LEMONGRASS	Electro-Magnetic Field Shield, Purifies Etheric, Repairs Auric Holes, Rat Race & Pressure, Pesky Irritations, Optimism, Courage to Overcome, Nervous System Calmed, Future Fears Eased	Purple, Red, Orange, Green
LEMON MYRTLE	Electro-Magnetic Fields, Light Assimilation & Aura Balancing, Male / Female Inner Balance, Resolve Internal Conflicts, Sumerian Past Lives, Past Life Secrets of Form & Nature	Greens, Gold, Pinks
LIME	Soothes Cellular Memories, Cleans, Joy, Revitalize, Karmic, Trauma, Etheric Salve, Lightness, Laughter, Inner Child & Body Issues, Cord Cut	Green, Gold, Blue, Magenta
NUTMEG	Betrayal & Loss Eased, Rigidity, Spontaneity, Flexibility, Detachment, New Foundations, Heart Dance With Joy, Connect To Wild & Free	Red, Orange, Yellow, Blue With Green Tinge, Purple
ORANGE SWEET	Purifies Emotional & Astral Body, Drama, Auric Density Eased, Repel Negative Entities, Judgmental-ism, Obsession	Purple, Silver-light, Gold, white

PALMAROSA	Divine Mother Energy, Love & Compassionate Acceptance, Role Models, Need To Be 'Perfect', Childhood, Abandonment	Magenta, Green Dark Yellow, Pinkish
PATCHOULI	Grounds, Will To Live, Growth/Change, Survival, Sexual Issues, Value Life, The 'Blues', Suicidal, Intimacy, Sensuality	Red/Orange, Violet Tinged With Purple-Gold Grounding
PEPPERMINT	Sacred Symbols & Geometry, Soul Truths, Higher Mind, For Terror, Hysteria, Fear of Unknown, Mind Chatter, Grounds 3rd Eye, Stomach, Resistance, Night Sweats	Pinks/ Greens, Metallic Blue, Silvery Light
PETITGRAIN	Overcome Obsessions & Addictions, Power Struggles, Internal Conflicts, Self Love, Acceptance, Anguish, Shame, Auric Rips, Heart Energy	Greenish-Yellow, Orange Grounding
ROSE OTTO	Rainbow Of Humanity, Unconditional Love, Relationships, Divine Stewardship, Transmute Burdens, Trust, Self Love, Soul Creativity, Inner Peace	Roman Pink, Teal Green to Blues, Gold & Silver
ROSEMARY	Soul Communication and Healing, Loyalty Discernment & Betrayal, Renewal, Recovery	Spring Green, Pearl-Silver, Royal-Blue to Peacock Blue
SAGE	DNA Codes, Ancestral Wisdom, Inadequacy, Self Judgment, Denial, Unfocused Direction, Self Sabotage, Needs, Expectations Of Others, Legs, Support, Oneness, Resourcefulness	Yellow Flame, Green, Silver, Electric Spectrum Orange
SANDALWOOD	Divine Sensuality, True Love, Sexuality, Calms Urges, Grounds, Kundalini	Orange-Pink, Purple, Green Grounding
YARROW	Psychic Protection, Wound Healer, Light Workers, Love & Clairvoyance, Ward Off Negativity, Enhance Clairvoyance, Seeking External Protection, Over-Sensitivity, Aura Compromise From Trauma Or Injury, Seals Energy Breaks In Aura, Overall Energy Fields Strengthener	Blue-Mauve Into Silver With Copper Hints, Moving Into Gold

| YLANGYLANG | Calm Nerves, Integrate Emotions, Fears, EMF, Revitalized, Anger, Frustration, Intimacy, Rejection, Jealousy, Boundaries, Own Destiny | Gold, Magenta, Green, Purple |

This Summary Chart is available in .pdf form to download and print out for genuine book buyers at http://www.myrasri.com/chart-for-book-buyers

<><><>

Myra Sri

INDIVIDUAL COLOUR CODES &
ACTIONS IN DEPTH

Descriptions of the Color Codes, their actions and effects energetically and etherically follows.

Usual Precautions (Unless Otherwise indicated):

Always use an Essential Oil diluted for topical skin application or massage. (Though in certain circumstances, Lavender Oil is generally safe for neat application.) Check on the purity of the oil as sometimes synthetics are used in inferior oil products. Always check on the purity of the oil when considering using orally, as few are of medicinal strength.

Illustrations:

The Author has attempted to convey some of the colours and etheric actions of some of the oils and has included them in colour in the ebook version.

If you would like to download the images from this book in colour, you can find them available for download at http://www.myrasri.com/chart-for-book-buyers

Glossary:

For your convenience there is a Glossary of Chakras and any bolded words at the end of the following section.

Further reading references also follow.

Layout

In an effort to assist easier reading and reference to the following information, opposite pages have been used wherever possible.

BASIL ESSENTIAL OIL

Basil helps to open pathways to Spiritual energy and our multi-dimensional consciousness to live more fully and so to manifest our desires or to be of service. Because it generates enthusiasm for life it allows us to release anxieties, restrictions or unwarranted inhibitions.

BENZOIN

Etheric Colours of Basil Essential Oil

Colour Codes; *Green, Coppery-Turquoise, Peacock Blue, Lavender, Silver-Tin*

The initial colour vibration of Green sets the space for nurture. This colour of nature allows space for the following burst of Coppery-Turquoise. The Turquoise aids inner dialogue between the self and spiritual communication and this is scattered with Copper Stars, which allows the opportunity to see more clearly on an inner level what needs to be dealt with.

As these Copper Stars combined with the Turquoise carries us through to the Peacock Blue scale of self trust and truth, this further enhances self confidence. Turquoise is a higher advanced colour code, and assists with spiritual communication and connection. The Peacock Blue gently opens us to inspiration.

Moving through this, we experience the first hint of red contained in the mauve-ish colour, which is combined with the Blue and White-Light to produce this mauve colour that settles to Lavender. This is the hint that activates and energizes, and also grounds the spiritual into the physical. The final sheen of Silver-Tin settles and seals the soul, bringing soothing spiritual comfort into the self and helps guide wiser actions.

Actions & Effects of Basil Essential Oil

Action Keywords; *Self Responsibility, Self-Esteem, Self-Judgment, Self-Limitation, Integrity, Spiritual Joy. Conscious Choices, Renewed Vitality. Manifestation. Brain Activation*

The actions of Basil Essential Oil directly impacts on the sinus cavities opening up the **Throat** Chakra. Working through the physical body to the **Base Chakra**, it helps anchor and ground for greater access by the **Higher Self** and the **Soul**.

A major action is its ability to support self responsibility and the true realities in one's life.

It is also known to be valuable for Sacro-Sexual-Spiritual balancing, working on harmonizing the 1st and 7th Chakras (**Base and Crown Chakras**). Bringing a more spiritual aspect to affect sexual impulses and safely assisting to address reasons behind sexual straying.

As outlined above in the Etheric colours section, we can follow how this enthuses and renews. As this oil initiates the space to review and re-choose past limits and old baggage, and helps provide a better higher connection, we can resurrect past goals or create higher goals that a previous low self view has hindered.

The Brain function is enhanced, aiding conscious choices that support the Self.

On the physical level, it is very invigorating and renewing, providing support when overcoming depression, anxiety, or doubts.

When light seekers are undergoing initiation or facing significant decisions, Basil generates comfort and encouragement.

More on Basil Essential Oil

Using diluted Basil on the gall bladder and liver meridians energetically supports the ability to be more responsible, and to assimilate life's inflow. Using it on the stomach meridian assists with self-trust and nourishment, and also easier relaxation. (The usual Dilution is 15-20 drops in 2 ounces of base oil. Always check for a reaction.)

This is a great oil to use on most meridians, and therapists can apply to acupressure points for quick effective energy relief.

Precautions:

Do not use on children or infants, and avoid during pregnancy. Diabetics should use with caution. As it can be irritating to the skin, avoid too much sun to avoid sensitizing.

BENZOIN ESSENTIAL OIL

I once heard this essential oil called the Oil of Abundance.

I do love the rich and luxurious bath that these energies give to the etheric body. And the sense of grounding and expansion that it brings.

Etheric Colours of Benzoin Essential Oil

Colour Codes; *Orange, Red, Deep Amber Gold with little Blue*

Benzoin launches into its etheric embrace with the colour code of Orange. This begins to work on our emotions, and any shock within the etheric body.

The focus into Red for vitality and life force then moves into the richness of Deep Amber Gold that bathes the etheric body, the emotional body, the astral body and strengthens the auric body.

As the Blue Glints bring a Bluish radiance to the Gold, the electromagnetic field is rebalanced and excess charge removed or settled. The electromagnetic aspect is recharged with a radiance that shuns any sense of lack.

Actions & Effects of Benzoin Essential Oil

Action Keywords; *Attracts, Soothe & Stimulate, Abundance, Depression*

The etheric actions of Benzoin's colour codes lifts the heavy energies associated with depression and thoughts of lack, and pulls in more etheric prana directly into the etheric field. This occurs whether you focus on inhaling or use the oil in massage, though the action is more intense with inhalation.

As it soothes and stimulates the etheric body and electromagnetic field, and bathes the senses with its rich, honeyed and sweet energy, its tendency to the attraction of abundance is easy to understand.

Working on the **Base Chakra, Sacral Chakra, Solar Plexus**, the **Third Eye Chakra**, and the **Navel Chakra**, it also connects in to the 2nd, 3rd, and 4th **Earthing Chakras**, as well as the **Link Chakra.**

The Governing meridian is assisted with this, so a back massage will surely bring benefit. Other meridians to benefit include the stomach, kidney, gall bladder and lung.

Its ability to ground in a sensual way is beautiful. For a beauty treatment or to feel treasured, to me, this is the 'chocolate' of essential oils.

More on Benzoin Essential Oil

Many, many years ago this oil had been recommended to me by someone who works with nature and the nature spirits, as well as being an international psychic. It took me ages to track it down, but its thick rich honeyed appearance and perfume were worth it. The aroma throughout my home was amazing!

It is also found in a specific massage oil blend and works well as such. It feels supportive and protective, as well as promoting that sense of being attractive and prosperous.

Used in certain 'rich' perfumes.

Bergamot Essential Oil

Used in Earl Grey tea, Bergamot is often produced in Italy, bringing a hint of the Mediterranean to some. Known as Bitter Orange, it is a powerful antiseptic in its own right, and can assist in allowing grace into one's life to encourage us to wholeness again.

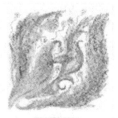

BERGAMOT

It is an emotional balancer and as a consequence, Judgments and restrictions are easier to deal with and to release.

Etheric Colours of Bergamot Essential Oil

Colour Codes; *Deep Greens, Deep Blues to Indigo, Bronze or Copper Feathered Magenta, Orange Spirals*

The initial wave of Deep Greens opens the Heart Chakra, allowing for greater love into the energy fields. As the Greens shift to Deep Blues the mind is toward calmness and peace and nervousness settles.

Oscillating into Indigo, our connection to the universal energies needed for spiritual growth is increased.

The etheric energies now create a wave of Magenta, which is feathered with Bronze or Copper sparks or twinkles. The twinkles activate the Solar Plexus and the Magenta stirs the Soul, which is supported with the Bronze and Copper. Copper supports the light bodies and the lower chakras.

Orange relieves held stress and soothes shock held in the etheric body, bathing the aura with its spirals.

Actions & Effects of Bergamot Essential Oil

Action Keywords;   *Opens The Heart, Calms Mental Body, Shock, Bitterness, Depression, Negative Thoughts, Power, Joy And Grace*

Opening to higher energies to help lift depressive and negative thoughts is a primary purpose of this oil. Issues of attachment, control, fear & trauma, depression, despair and guilt can be addressed and soothed, or released and healed if that is the intent.

Bergamot oil aids to address long held or unsupportive beliefs & emotions, and programmed tendencies toward resistance, calming the mental body. The action allows for despair and guilt to open to joy and serenity and grace. This can aid in a renewal of enthusiasm again.

It works by expanding the **Heart Chakra**, and the **Solar Plexus** then aligns to assist to overcome power or control issues. This calms the mental body, whilst cellular memory from the physical body is more easily accessed and cleared. Shock and stress is eased allowing for recovery and healing.

The **Soul** becomes more fully aligned. Joy and grace are more abundant.

Bergamot can assist with resetting the body's thermostat energetically via the thyroid. And also assist to restore balance to it again.

More on Bergamot Essential Oil

Dense energy in the Solar Plexus can be transmuted, aligning it with the heart. Bergamot can cool an excess heat that is held in the body. Encourages the light bodies to assimilate energy better.

The Chakras that respond best are the **Heart, Navel** and **Solar Plexus Chakras**.

The gall bladder meridian, central, spleen and bladder meridians all benefit with this oil.

Precautions:

Avoid use before sun-tanning in the sun or on a sunbed. Once used for sun preparations to assist in faster tanning, it was found to increase photosensitivity of the skin, causing burning.

CAJEPUT ESSENTIAL OIL

Emotional dysfunction regarding sexual roles, and the patterns from inappropriate gender role models are addressed. Initially for some, this oil can seem harsh or simply not pleasant, whereas to others its aroma may be perceived and experienced as sharp, crisp and uplifting.

It brings fresh energy into resolving relationships.

Etheric Colours of Cajeput Essential Oil

Colour Codes; *Orange-InfraRed, Silver, Green Spectrum*

Orange Light is the initial etheric emergence, quickly joined with a Pillar Box InfraRed. InfraRed activates the etheric body to release cellular memories of disharmony which need to be dealt with. These two forces of Orange Light and InfraRed now merge into spirals of colour codes that also combine to deliver the soothing qualities of Coral. These three actions work on issues of relationships, unrequited love, imbalances in having a healthy rapport between desire and the intimacy of true love.

Fading into Silvery threads, the action moves to the **Soul** area. The materialization of the Green Spectrum flame now brings a greater connection between heart, desire, emotions, life force and soul.

Actions & Effects of Cajeput Essential Oil

Action Keywords; *Dysfunctional /Abusive Relationships, Male Traits of Control, Domination Integrates To Receptivity, Fulfill Own Needs, Sexual Issues, Inertia, Self Expression, True Spiritual Love*

The imbalances of being either too male or too female can be addressed, encouraging one to support both their inner male and their inner female. In particular, domination by males can be viewed differently, as the hardened layers of self protection soften and the encrusting loosens to allow for the release of the childhood or past life issues, memories and patterns that have been inherited or brought through.

Encompassing the **Root Chakra, Sacral Chakra, Solar Plexus, Heart Chakra, Throat Chakra** and the little known **Sex Chakra** in its effectual embrace, Cajeput brings tempering, awareness, greater true self-expression and joy of enhanced relating into one's life experience.

Because of this essential oil's action on these Chakras, the Soul is willing to explore this area more readily. During healing energy work, this can be extremely helpful, as it can go where other modalities cannot reach.

The Thyroid is also supported, and energetic distortions or debris that suppress self-esteem can release. Self expression in sexual intimacy becomes easier and more free and freeing.

More on Cajeput Essential Oil

Can assist with Past Life issues, especially where there has been chauvinism, misogyny, sexual bigotry or prejudice, either experienced or perpetrated.

Use as massage on the throat and womb area in women in those cases of hysterectomy, or to help with suppressed sexual issues. Massaged into the gall bladder meridian it can assist with cellular memories of abuse. Lung meridians for sorrow or stress, the heart meridian and back or Governing meridian for self doubt and hurt.

Apply to the **4 ½ point Chakra** for releasing drains to others who are close to you.

Precautions:

Do not use with children of any age. Always check for purity with this oil as it is often diluted with synthetics. Take the usual precautions.

Carnation Essential Oil

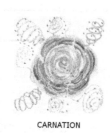

CARNATION

Carnation speaks directly of **Past Lives** and previous incarnations. It is protective, and allows for access to those times hidden behind 'the veil', as well as issues that are triggered by Past Life events, memories or imprints.

Past life issues often involve inter-dimensional frequencies and domains, which do require some knowledge and navigating and often need a degree of ethical and energetic understanding to manage safely.

This oil can aid in these travels as it is grounding and protective.

Etheric Colours of Carnation Essential Oil

Colour Codes; *Rich Pink-Mauve, Blue, Gold-Silver with Green Flecks*

The Rich Pink-Mauve is a variation of Magenta, bringing more of the frequency of White-Light to aid purification.

It begins its work by bringing more gentleness and peace to the **Base** Chakra, aligning it with the **Heart** Chakra, and the **Crown** Chakra. As the heart begins to balance to more acceptance of one's current incarnation, its light tends to shine more clearly.

Having established the Pink aspects of this etheric code, the Mauve tends and trends to clear Blue tendrils which works on bringing to consciousness issues of expression and stimulates the Thymus. The **Throat Chakra** begins to clear, and The **Soul Seat**, which sits etherically behind or near the Thymus is stimulated.

With this activation, the spirals of Gold Silver now emanating from Carnation oil now spirals, trickling into the chakras together with Green Flecks. This combination works towards strengthening and healing the **Soul** and **Major Chakras.**

Actions & Effects of Carnation Essential Oil

Action Keywords; *Protection, Past Life and Reincarnation Issues, Soul Memories, Life Force, Grounding, Emotional Objectivity, Learning, Focus*

This is power oil. Great for restoring energy and life force.

Carnation (Absolute) Essential Oil stimulates & cleanses the entire auric field & strengthens the aura. It also helps to rid the aura of negative Thoughtforms.

Because of its grounding abilities and capacity to connect with the **Higher Chakras,** the Soul, other dimensions and the **New Earthing Chakras,** it aids Past Life regressions or healings. The Soul is more ready to receive if there is a lesson to be had, or to understand and resolve in a more receptive way.

The **Earthing Chakras** 5th and 8th benefit from using this oil, as it works to resolve previous incarnational experiences as other consciousnesses.

Many have directly chosen their family or parents in this incarnation, and this oil assist alignment with ancestral chi and planetary Earth chi. This is linked to the kidney meridian, and small intestine meridian, both related to nourishment and family. The Governing meridian also benefits.

More on Carnation Essential Oil

Though not always easy to find, this oil is well worth having in your kit. Because it can also work with ley-lines, it is great to have around for an energy builder of stamina.

CEDARWOOD ESSENTIAL OIL

Cedarwood essential oil stimulates the ability to connect with hope and faith again, as it tends to open up energy constrictions and allow a feeling of security through. The subtle bodies are brought back into balance or alignment, and energy can flow more easily through them.

Etheric Colours of Cedarwood Essential Oil

Colour Codes; *Blue, Opalescent Blue-Green Tinged With Deep Orange & Purple*

This is a complicated array of codes. Beginning with Blue as the first etheric colour, Cedarwood then moves into its Opalescent Blue-Green frequency, which addresses the emotions and old situations, whilst bringing spiritual energy through immediately. The ability to see within and to see under our feelings assists with accepting the true reality, and not just what we think we see.

The emergence of the Deep Orange tips and Purple tinges helps to bring more lightness whilst lightening our attitudes and our 'load'.

One feels more protected as stress and anxiety are sifted and the mind becomes clearer and calmer.

Actions & Effects of Cedarwood Essential Oil

Action Keywords; *Security & Protection, Clarity, Focus, Direction, Dispel Fantasy Projections, Energy Flow, True Spiritual Love, Hope & Faith for Hearts Desires*

Cedarwood brings clarity and the energy to dispel illusions. This creates a space for re-assessing direction and also seeing reality how it is and accepting is. Love is more easily recognized as the acceptance it really is, and that it is already present. Finding our love within can help us fulfill desires without the illusions of lust or over romanticized ideals, and to recognize the spirit within others.

Stress is eased in the mental and physical body, and inhaling it helps to slow down and relax the mind too busy with analysis. Energy flows more easily and brings with it a more spiritual tone.

Cedarwood activates and stimulates the **Heart Chakra, Throat Chakra** and **Sacral Chakra**. It also connects in with the **Higher Chakras**. This connects us to knowing more of our aspects, and the cause of our needs.

Most meridian applications benefit from this essential oil and its etheric actions. The kidney meridian settles ancestral patterns related to mistrust and fear. Applying to the heart meridian helps to release the need for substitutes for love. Large intestine assists release and flow, and the gall bladder meridian supports toxin release. The liver meridian is good for overall integration.

More on Cedarwood Essential Oil

Cedarwood is also cleansing & protective. Good for troubled dreams & children's sleep. Sometimes used in furniture polishes, it can bring a comforting and more 'real' sense to the home.

Take the usual precautions.

<><><>

CHAMOMILE ESSENTIAL OIL

It is generally known that Chamomile calms, but not how. The frequencies of Chamomile promote peace and help to sedate the nervous system, soothing heartache and hurt around love issues. Intuition is more easily accessed as is inner reconnection.

Etheric Colours of Chamomile Essential Oil

Colour Codes; *Turquoise, Bluish-Purple, Iridescent Green, Gold, Silver, White*

The initial experience of Chamomile is the Turquoise frequency. This takes us to within our self from focus on the external, opening us to inner communication.

From here, we trend to the blue aspect, moving into a Bluish-Purple, similar to Royal Blue-Indigo. This frequency assists with inner vision or intuition, and resonates at the **Causal Chakra**. The colour vibrations align us to more of our own power as well as more receptivity to divine will and timing.

Iridescent Green further calms body, mind and Soul, furthering our connection to Divine Source. There is an etheric green cube usually situated within the trunk of the body that this colour code re-aligns for present timing on the physical, soul and mental dimensions. This helps to anchor us back into the 'Now'.

When Gold and Silver combine with our etheric fields, we experience strength, support, connection and Soul soothing. Our auric field is loved and soothed as well as our nervous system and mind.

White-Light then further enhances the detoxification of negativity on any level, slowing through to assist with purifying the etheric body.

Actions & Effects of Chamomile Essential Oil

Action Keywords; *Calms Conscious Mind, Peace, Anger, Loneliness, Abandonment, Grief, Nervous System, Stress, Death Wishes, Heartbreak, Lost Love, Divine Right Timing, Life Transitions, Ghosts*

Issues of abandonment, loneliness, buried anger and or grieving as well as death wishes can be relieved as the etheric liver and nervous system greatly benefits from this soothing oil. The personality becomes clearer and lighter from its load, and beliefs can be re-assessed. Its processes are all gentle, and they bring the space to nurse oneself through the pain without the usual associated intensity.

The energy between spirit and material matter is eased and balanced. Any self hate or disgust can be alleviated, and more regard for self can come through.

Intense experiences can be soothed, giving easier introspection into traumatic or dramatic events.

The **Heart Chakra** is widely expanded, the **Causal Chakra** is balanced, the etheric nervous system and most of the organs are supported and eased, and a gentle detoxification shifts how one sits within the body.

The Governing meridian helps overcoming fears around living and dying. Central meridian benefits when there are fears of separation from Divine Source. These two govern the tone of the meridian system. In fact, apply anywhere and everywhere the body feels that it needs it, as it will work meta-physically to support any related issue that is indicating itself physically. Your body will know, so listen to it!

The **Soul** feels nurtured, and more hope for living, and ease for the dying occurs.

More on Chamomile Essential Oil

It has been said that everybody needs chamomile and that the body absolutely loves it! When researched, it has been discovered that this oil, when taken as a form of tea, greatly feeds and supports the harmony of the subtle bodies, particularly in the digestive and nervous system. This is why it is highly recommended in tea form. In essential oil form, it is indeed powerful.

Transition over to the other side is assisted with Chamomile essential oil. It can be used in meditation, prayer or invocation to call on angelic help – infuse or inhale to make the connection – as it helps to open to the Angelic Realms who can further assist with their help in clearing earth bound entities that are trying to attach, or souls fearful of passing over.

It is also helpful when experiencing the loss of someone and very consoling when used during the grieving period.

Anywhere on the body is helped with Chamomile. The body loves it, and may even crave it for a while after if there is a need for this oil once the body has been introduced to it.

Secrets Beyond Aromatherapy

CINNAMON ESSENTIAL OIL

Cinnamon Bark & Cinnamon Leaf

Though generally the Etheric Colours and actions of Cinnamon Leaf and Cinnamon Bark are similar, it is worth noting a couple of differences in their actions.

CINNAMON

The leaf tends to support the aura and electromagnetic energy systems, whereas the bark tends to act in a deeper and more physical way, particular on the nervous system and digestive system.

The actual pod or 'fruit' of the Cinnamon in the form we can buy in supermarkets and shops can work on both the circulatory system and the digestive system. However, the essential oil is a much more concentrated form of vitality and can work not only physically and energetically but also etherically. Etheric action includes the Light Bodies as well as the chakras, and can work inter-dimensionally. Energetic action includes the meridian systems of the body, the energy flow between the chakras, and any action causing the moving or releasing of energy blockages.

Etheric Colours of Cinnamon Essential Oil

Colour Codes; Red, Green, Orange, Blue

The igniting and vitalizing effect of Red on the etheric and energy bodies begins the process of activating the energy necessary for change. A bold essence, it also grounds and centers the body. Releasing a life-force fire, it then moves into its opposite in the colour spectrum to:

This now brings nurturing into the picture. Green is a combination of Blue and Yellow, and as such works on the mental body, the will and identity aspects and the expression chakra at the throat.

Maintaining the yellow ray hidden in green, the etheric colour then moves into the Orange side of the colour spectrum, providing emotional containment, and countering the tendency to depression, inviting one to step into life again. The shift continues with the move to its almost opposite in the spectrum again -

The energetic actions now begin to settle into Blues, light and mid-Blue through to royal Blue, the result here being a protective sealing and assurance, and a return to a sense of one's own inner truth. Communication on the inner level is activated.

Actions & Effects of Cinnamon Essential Oil

Action Keywords; *Transitions, Past Life Healing, Cellular Memory, Victim and Enslavement Issues, Power, Abuse, Dogma.* <u>*Related Issues*</u>: *Anger, Abundance, Lack of Happiness, Attachments*

Cinnamon is quite fiery in that it can assist with the release of long held or forgotten memories related to abuse, power, slavery or trauma. It can bring these things up for awareness and release, whether related to this life or from a Past life. Cellular memories are contacted and brought up for healing.

If you are in the process of creating change in your life, then Cinnamon can give the motivating force, and assist you particularly with allowing new attitudes and new responses. Dogma and restrictions are addressed, and the fears and patterns associated with them can be reviewed.

When using Cinnamon oil for self healing, be aware that you will be in a process of releasing energy that had previously been trapped and so remember to remind yourself not to get caught up in the old energies being released. Rather, note what you are experiencing, and stay in present time, and if necessary breathe through the uncomfortable parts, focusing instead on the beauty of the colour code, and in creating the new. You may even choose to follow it up with another essential oil such as Lavender, Rose or Orange.

Enslavements from the past are more easily transformed to freedom, and more abundance can be embraced when working with this oil. Particularly when used in a carrier oil and applied to the **Base Chakra**. This technique can also generate more vitality, and will for life. But use it wisely and sparingly in this area. Monitor its effects and also check the **Precautions** section.

When applied to the heart area, it can allow the heart to cope with change and enhance feelings of security with the self.

Besides being used for **Soul** Healing, and Emotional balancing, Cinnamon essential oil may promote physical energy, psychic awareness, and assist in increasing one's prosperity.

Cellular memory over power issues can be more easily accessed and released. Issues of anger, abuse, frustration or attachment can become more settled when addressed consciously using this oil with aware and conscious Breathing.

Chakras that benefit or are activated with Cinnamon are: **Base Chakra**, **Sacral Chakra**, **Navel Chakra**, **Heart Chakra**, **Crown Chakra** and the **5th Earthing Chakra**.

Meridians supported are circulation-sex, triple warmer, heart and small intestine. Working on these assists with feelings of insecurity in relationships, and assists with releasing old patterns. Used on the kidney meridian assists with feelings of mistrust, anxiety and fear, and can further assist the adrenals.

Cinnamon Health Benefits and More

Cinnamon supports the 'Fire' element noted in TCM in the physical body due to this action and enhancement in digestion. But in the etheric body, it has an emotionally warming lunar energy and is more aligned with the 'Water' element', thus allowing for introspection and insight. Lunar energy is connected with the changing and shifting emotions, a condition of human life. Using Lunar energy in etheric healing like this assists in going with the flow.

Studies have found that Cinnamon supplement may have a beneficial effect on blood sugar, and it may be because Cinnamon contains a good amount of chromium, an essential trace mineral that helps in the action of insulin.

Cinnamon has been used for treating rheumatism and other inflammations. Cinnamon has antibacterial and antifungal properties. It's active against Candida albicans, the fungus that causes yeast infections and thrush, and Helicobacter pylori, the bacteria responsible for stomach ulcers.

Cinnamon extracts can also inhibit the growth of cultured tumor cells. This effect may be due to the presence of procyanidins and eugenol in the bark extract.

Cinnamon is also useful as a food preservative to inhibit the growth of common food-borne bacteria such as Salmonella and E coli. Adding a sprinkle to your meals is an easy way to take Cinnamon and even using it in a stir fry it is often masked with other flavors. One way of including it in your diet is to mix it with honey, and use as a breakfast spread on your toast. Don't overdo it, as this oil *can* be overdone.

Precautions:

Taking Cinnamon supplement together with the diabetes medication or any medication can make blood glucose levels dip too low. Cassia Cinnamon in supplement form naturally contains a compound called coumarin. At very high levels, coumarin may damage the liver. Coumarin can also have a 'blood-thinning' effect, so nutritional supplements should **not** be taken by people with bleeding disorders or who take prescription anti-clotting medication. **Always** seek your doctor's approval before taking Cinnamon supplement.

Most concentrated Cinnamon oils are not intended for consumption, but instead are used for aromatherapy essential oils. This oil is very strong and an overdose may depress the central nervous system. One should not take the oil to treat a condition unless under the supervision of a health care expert.

Pregnant women are advised to avoid taking Cinnamon oil or large doses of the bark, since high doses may induce abortion.

<><><>

Secrets Beyond Aromatherapy

CITRONELLA ESSENTIAL OIL

Most people are aware of using Citronella for deterring mosquitoes and flies, but not for use as an essential oil.

Citronella is good for bacteria, acting as an anti-viral. This is very useful around coughs, colds or similar symptoms. On a basic etheric level, it aids in grounding and anchoring.

Etheric Colours of Citronella Essential Oil

Colour Codes: *Tannish-Orange Tinged Red, Yellow*

Tannish-Orange, Tinged Red: This interesting mix of colours tends to speak of a simmering earthy type of infra-red. The centre of the etheric impulse has a grounded heart which emanates outward to a protective Red tinged flare that also provides forward vitality. This then is absorbed to stabilize the physical body and to ground the emotional body leading to:

Yellow is generally considered to balance the mental body, but here it also addresses the nervous system in order to bring greater clarity. From a grounded perspective, space is gained to view more positive alternatives.

Actions & Effects of Citronella Essential Oil

Action Keywords: *Nervous System, Sugar Imbalances/ Lost Joy, Quick Anger, Comfort & Courage to Resolve Conflicts*

As can be seen by the etheric colour language, this little known or uncommon essential oil is quite powerful. Red has been associated with anger, but here the energy is more emotionally grounded enabling the spiky Reds in the aura caused by anger outbursts or tendencies to settle.

The **Sacral Chakra** is balanced in a grounded way, aiding courage and providing comfort. The flow on to the Yellow allows for the calming of anger, in a positive manner, and the opportunity to learn to use anger in a constructive way.

It can assist with sugar imbalances – the cause is often the loss of joy which can lead to a lack of sweetness in life or the inability to recognize and utilize joy that is already present.

Sugar consumption or overload 'hits' only further stir up and overload the adrenals. Citronella can aid to further reduce the need for sugar through avoiding interpersonal confrontation and assist in finding a resolution with a more balanced nervous system. The **Throat Chakra** is also assisted.

It would appear that not only physical viruses and infections can be tackled with Citronella, but it can also address etheric viruses and provide clarity. As well as supporting the immune system, on a metaphysical level it will also support one's energetic defense systems, giving anchoring, comfort and access to more enjoyment.

Energetic Parasitic energies can be addressed with Citronella. Like Lemongrass, it helps to repel these tiny multiple invaders, which always show in the etheric body before gaining a hold on the physical body.

Citronella supports the spleen, triple-warmer and large intestine meridians to enhance the immune system. Used on the heart, gall bladder and kidney, it assists with reducing pessimism and anger.

More on Citronella Essential Oil

There is not much more to be added at this point, as we are still learning about this delightfully unassuming oil.

Though I can further add that even when not deliberately working or applying it energetically, it has been found that when combining with Orange it gives a pleasant mental lift, particularly when one is working at a computer.

As mentioned earlier, it is also useful for deterring insects as well as most mosquitoes at night.

TIPS

STATEMENTS FOR MAJOR **MERIDIANS**:

Central Meridian:

    I respect myself

    I respect those that deserve respect

Governing Meridian:

    I have support

    I easily support myself

    I accept my feelings

Heart Meridian:

    I love and accept myself

    I am tolerant of myself and others

    I love and accept others wisely

CLARY SAGE ESSENTIAL OIL

Clary Sage essential oil is great for quietening the chatter of the mind. It also aids focus, and on a practical level, supports study. Clarity is restored, and the heavy energies around the head can clear.

Overly Sensitive types may need to use this in combination with another oil as it is very effective for bringing in a high degree of expansion and high level energies. See Precaution notes below.

Etheric Colours of Clary Sage Essential Oil

Colour Codes; *Deep Blue, Gold becoming Transparent Gold, Pearlised Yellow, Magenta*

The vibration of Deep Blue initiates peace within the body and being. Resistance is eased and change is allowed in.

The grounding depth and glorious shimmer of Gold now connects us to the higher spiritual planes, and strengthens our etheric and auric fields. This Golden frequency shifts to a Transparent version, leaving the film of Gold as the etheric vibrations allow for another octave into the frequencies.

The colour vibration now moves into a Pearlised Yellow that shimmers like the glow of a yellow pearl. Pearl is about kindness to one's self, and Pearlised Yellow is the frequency of kindness and clarity within the mind.

Moving into Magenta, the entire energy system is nurtured and the etheric is protected. The power of Magenta helps to kind of 'lock-in' these gained benefits. The symbol associated with the action of this oil is the square; representing stability.

Actions & Effects of Clary Sage Essential Oil

Action Keywords; *Stops Mind Chatter, Stillness Of Joy, Mental Focus, Confusion, Paranoia, Obsessive Thoughts,*

Dense Energy Of Depression/ Sorrow, Burdens, Crisis, Anguish / Anxiety, Kidney/ Lungs

As with most essential oils, there is an aspect of the spiritual, no matter that many use them for physical or emotional benefits. This is the case here, with Clary Sage.

Its ability to calm, quieten and still the mind and its chatter is remarkable. It eases and even lifts depression and sorrow, anguish and anxiety, and removes dense energies from around the head and heart.

The etheric body is eased, and the kidneys function more easily, allowing for a better degree of hydration. This further assists the brain and mind. Obsessive thoughts can be cleared as Thoughtforms of confusion that have depleted the energy and vitality now clear. Paranoia and the tendency to crisis can be addressed as patterns can be more easily seen.

Third Eye Chakra, Throat Chakra, Heart Chakra, Navel Chakra, the new **Psychic Body Chakras**, the etheric body, the crystalline light body and the following meridians benefit from the clearing that occurs with Clary Sage: lung, triple warmer, bladder, large intestine, gall bladder, stomach and kidney.

More on Clary Sage Essential Oil

Used before a test, this oil enhances and stimulates a clear mental state and energizes thinking. Easily inhaled before study or examinations, you can easily carry it in a pocket. If you are sensitive, use another oil after the test/exam to bring you more fully back into your normal mode (and to be more grounded).

Massaged into the entire Solar Plexus area, it helps to clear out depression and sorrow as it hits on several meridians and organs.

Precautions:

If you are very sensitive and are possibly likely to experience too much joy and euphoria, ensure you also use a grounding oil with Clary Sage to assist you to function on the practical and physical again. If you experience an out of body occurrence, use something like Clove, Juniper, Patchouli, Carnation, Fennel, Lemongrass, Sandalwood or Yarrow. Even though I have not yet written about Vetivert, this is also a positive support for grounding too.

In the unlikely but possible event you experience a headache, drink more water and use a grounding oil as above. It will pass quickly, and you will feel a lot lighter than before you used Clary Sage. The pain is usually simply held in toxins being released quickly as your energy field expands and expels.

CLOVE ESSENTIAL OIL

Clove often reminds one of Christmas time and Christmas pudding or cake, especially when blended with Cinnamon and Nutmeg oils, and sometimes Lime.

Clove Oil has been aptly described as 'the velvet covered hammer'... aiding self-expression whilst releasing Auric density and emotions related to abuse.

The mouth and teeth also benefit from this oil, and it was used in times gone by for mouth and teeth problems as well as to treat pain.

Etheric Colours of Clove Bud

Colour Codes; *Orange, Red, Mauve / Violet, Violet tinged with Teal and Gold*

We begin with Orange, which is great for any sort of shock, or loss of joy. Working initially on the Sacral Chakra, which is located between the groin and the belly button, it assists in bringing the emotional body back into alignment. Usually shock causes a shift, if not a displacement, of the emotional etheric body. The saying 'I was beside-myself' describes this displacing accurately. Having balanced this area, the energetic action moves on to:

Red is not only a grounding colour, it is also a protective colour. As the Sacral chakra rebalances, and the emotional body comes back into the body, there can be a reconnection back to that which 'blew' the fuse in the first place. Here the Red grounds and provides vitality to move through the issue, the colour now progressing to:

Mauve / Violet: Now we begin the connection with the spiritual aspects again, the higher strengths. Mauve enlivens the spiritual body, whilst the Violet transmutes negativity and negative energies.

Next, we have the Violet tinged with Teal and Gold: Violet intensifies, connecting the central Chakra Core between both Base chakra and Crown chakra. Teal now shows in the perimeter of the colour, blending with Golden layers. The Teal allows re-centering back into the heart and its

Blue aspect strengthens the connection to the Throat chakra for better self expression.

Actions & Effects of Clove Bud

Action Keywords; *Auric Clearing, Emotional Re-Connection, Root Of Pain, Self Expression, Shock, Gentle Power, Kundalini, Joy, Grounding*

The action of Clove is essentially to enhance the right use of the energy of power, tempering it with gentleness. To do so, it needs to clear any misuse of power. And any associated shock, whether the misuse is by one's self or experienced at the hands of another. In this way, anger is also moved out of the aura.

It also assists in moving any blocked Kundalini energy out through the mouth and throat.

The sequencing of the colours assists in recognizing our denials, rigidities, and defensiveness and the pains that may have caused them. It also allows for tranquility and therefore the space to reconnect spiritually.

Another benefit of the colour codes of Clove Bud is the transformation of self-consciousness into a practical use of the underlying blocked creative forces. Self-expression is encouraged, and patterns of self-consciousness are eased.

Chakras affected and supported by Clove are: **Base Chakra, Sacral Chakra, Throat Chakra, Crown Chakra** and the Soles of the **Feet.**

Meridians that are supported with Clove are: stomach, spleen, bladder, gall bladder and Governing.

More on Clove Bud Essential Oil

It has often long been connected on the physical level with reducing pain of toothache, and for problems with the Teeth, Mouth and Throat. Often this sort of pain is merely a symptom of repression. Dealing with the problem on an energetic and etheric level will greatly enhance and amplify the possible physical benefits of this oil and its amazing array of glorious colours.

Teeth often represent our ability to 'chew' life over, or lets us know if we have 'bitten' off more than we can handle (or 'chew'), as well as when things are 'gnawing' at us. Childhood issues can often affect the teeth, as the teeth and jaw can also represent strength, which can be affected if one has experienced terror.

The jaw can hold anger and repressed emotions which will create problems in one's 'bite'. This inner tension can translate into a violent outburst of some kind, whether internally toward one's self, or externally towards others. There may be bursts of anger, whether public or hidden in private. Releasing this internal pressure will benefit the whole of the mouth, jaw and neck area, and help release old fear.

Fennel Essential Oil

The liquorice type scent of Fennel Essential Oil immediately engages the senses and triggers off connections with food, the thyroid, yummy eating memories and related subconscious associations. A sense of satisfaction seems to accompany Fennel. This delicious oil will help where there has been the feeling of lack in life.

Etheric Colours of Fennel Essential Oil

Colour Codes; *Yellow/Lemon, Coppery-Green, Light Green, Soft Infra Tiny Stars in Clear/Transparent*

Lemon-Yellow is the first spiral of etheric energy, bringing the possibility of clarity at the sense doors, and allowing for fluency and accuracy within the intellect. As it moves on to spirals of the Coppery-Green, our connection to nature expands and the bright transition metal of Copper provides possibilities of new re-wiring to further support this. As Light Green begins to create more freshness and space for one's inner truth, the oil re-ignites then anchors the present time flow within the upper torso. This can ease the breath.

Next, there is a wave of clear transparent energy, scattered with tiny reddish Stars which appear like an Infrared frequency, but is a lot more calming. This stimulates further available healing energy and a better grasp of Nurturing Chi, whilst providing grounding for the spiritual as well as physical aspects.

This promises well for those desiring to change habits.

Actions & Effects of Fennel Essential Oil

Action Keywords; *Fears Of Lack, Substituting Food Or Other Substances For Love, Weight Issues, Self-Rejection, Thyroid, Self-Nourishment, Past Life Experiences Of Famine, Survival Or Weight And Power Associations*

The etheric thyroid can be stimulated with Fennel, with insecurity and control issues surfacing to be released. Weight issues, whether overeating or anorexic type tendencies, and the related holding on to hurts can be addressed. Past life memories where weight was revered as power, or where famine issues existed may surface. Mediterranean cultures, Egyptian lifetimes connected with the Goddess Isis may also be recovered in certain types of therapy.

It works on these **Major Chakras: - Base Chakra**, the **Solar Plexus** and the **Heart Chakra**, the **Crown Chakra** and also the New **Earthing Chakras.**

More on Fennel Essential Oil

Fennel opens us up to spiritual self-love needed to overcome fears around self-image, lack, and bottled up emotions causing weight issues.

It is highly recommended for meridian massage or even general all over massage where there are weight issues.

Massaging into certain meridians can unblock energy. In a carrier oil (15 drops to 2 ounces of base oil) massage into the large intestine and stomach meridian to promote self-trust and self-nourishment. Massage into the gall bladder meridian to assist with energy blocks and to support fat metabolism.

Precautions:

Avoid during pregnancy. Also if there is any epilepsy. Care when using with children.

FRANKINCENSE ESSENTIAL OIL

Frankincense is commonplace in some churches and meditation centers, and it is often commonly used for dynamic purification and cleansing of the aura. For those with negative church-type associations connected with this oil,

FRANKINCENSE

please do not let that prevent you from taking advantage of this complicated, yet highly effective oil.

Through the way it works on the chakras and light body, Frankincense can help to awaken us to our spiritual integrity, purpose and responsibility. It can also open doors to other realms of consciousness and helps to increase spiritual growth.

It can also assist us to see our obsessions.

Etheric Colours of Frankincense Essential Oil

Colour Codes; *Silver-Gold Yellow turning into Silvery Mauve/Blue with deep Blue Flame*

Initiating with Silver-Gold, these two metallic colours oscillate, strengthening the auric bodies, upper or Higher chakras. They then condense, eventuating into a Silvery Mauve ray that holds a Deep Blue Flame within. The Blue relates to honesty, truth and divine protection. On the mental level it can activate correct thinking.

On other levels, it can assist with honest introspection, higher visions and aid in crossing time barriers.

The effect is profound, as all of these colours contain spiritual intent. The Gold stimulates regeneration and the Silver eases nervous tension.

The Deep Blue Flame also assists with anchoring resonations to the new Human **Earthing Chakras** that are evolving in these times.

Actions & Effects of Frankincense Essential Oil

Action Keywords; *Spiritual Purpose, Growth & Choice, Denial, Life Force, Integrity, Mastery, Soul Memories, I Am, Serenity*

Frankincense appears to increase oxygenation energetically. The life force is enlarged physically and etherically. The etheric colours affect the following **Chakras: Crown, Third Eye, Heart** and also the Light Body. New dimensions can be accessed, as can ancient memories when meditating or working energetically.

Soul memories can be retrieved, and patience can be accessed.

Serenity can enter the soul, and used in meditation or with intent, can help one connect with their Divine essence.

Massage along the liver and spleen meridians to integrate, energize and balance the body and being. When massaged into the kidney area, it can help to ground the body into the present whilst also assisting with strengthening one's spiritual purpose. Used on the heart meridian can remind one of their spiritual path and pursuit.

More on Frankincense Essential Oil

When someone is going through transitions in life, using the oil on the heart meridian, as well as the large intestine, lung and triple heater meridians will make the change easier. This facilitates better and greater use of Prana.

Physical terrors may be eased by massaging along the Conception (or Central) Meridian and the Governing Meridian. These are major controllers in the etheric energy flow within the in-body chakras.

Secrets Beyond Aromatherapy

GARDENIA ESSENTIAL OIL

This sweet perfumed oil is not always easy to track down, but worth is certainly the effort. Gardenia helps to support the etheric body and is valuable when one is constantly around a lot of people, particular those with problems. Found in certain perfumes, it has a pleasant charming aroma with a hint of honey and warm evenings.

Etheric Colours of Gardenia Essential Oil

Colour Codes; *Blue, Mauve/Purple, Gold, Opalescent Pink*

Gardenia's etheric codes are quite pretty. The initial Blue oscillations from the oil now gives way to tones of pink and blue, manifesting as Mauve. This is accompanied with Purple twinkle type glints.

This colour combination process first brings in more peace into the energy fields, then a sense of benevolence. As it turns to Mauve and its Purple hints, another dimension opens to attract more light that supports the mental body, the emotional body and the etheric body.

As the glory of Gold emerges into the colour play, it opens the Core of the Being to its own resources. This supports the energy fields in expansion and vibrational integrity of the aura.

The gentle pulse of Opalescent Pink now takes centre stage, and soothes the heart area and the Soul, whilst bathing the outer aura with a gentle coating of this glimmering Pink. This can now gently assist those others who are around this gentle colour towards self calming.

Actions & Effects of Gardenia Essential Oil

Action Keywords; *Peace, Attract Good Vibrations*

Overall this is an oil of 'feel-good' and peace.

Gardenia can help to prevent energy drains as the energy fields move into a space that supports auric awareness and wholeness. The actions of Gardenia etheric colours and vibrations help to strengthen the aura.

When one is around disruptive people and situations, it also helps to stabilize the aura. Because of its qualities it can bring a calming effect into the immediate area. After a few minutes this oil can help to calm others, as the opalescent qualities combined with the pink attract more love and light into the space.

As it helps to repel negativity, it is a great essential oil for counselors, as well as other 'people people' such as healers, practitioners, nurses and psychics etc.

The Chakras that benefit from Gardenia essential oil are: the **Heart Chakra, Causal Chakra** and **Third Eye Chakra.**

The new Chakra Systems also are assisted to align and integrate with the Major Chakra Systems to, especially the **Psychic Body Chakras,** the **Link Chakra** and **Navel Chakra.**

Central and Governing meridians, and the heart are supported with Gardenia. This helps bring 'tone' to the entire meridian system.

More on Gardenia Essential Oil

The effect of Gardenia is generally to 'feel-good' – it doesn't make you want to jump for joy, or race out and change the world, but it does make you easier to get along with to others, and for you, it makes getting along with others easier. And today, with so much sense of separation and lack of support, this is a good thing.

Precautions:

Take the usual precautions. Get the best quality you can.

GERANIUM ESSENTIAL OIL

Keywords for Rose Geranium are centered around actions of nurturing, balancing, soothing and feelings of safety.

Often a commonplace plant in most gardens, the scent is very familiar.

Etheric Colours of Geranium Essential Oil

Colour Codes; *Pink-Green, Gold*

The **Heart Chakra** is the first to feel the impact of Geranium's etheric colours of Pink-Green. Green is the common heart space colour, and the Pink is the new and recent Heart opener vibration. Together, they bring the physical heart and the 'higher' heart of universality into harmony and alignment.

These combine as the '**Twin Hearts**' and set off a series of activations within the whole of the Chakra system.

Gold then follows this powerful combination to further strengthen the activities and processes already set in place. This allows for the **Soul** to be strengthened and supported, and the light bodies to vibrate to a higher frequency. Not only does this activate more love, it also strengthens the connection with one's Divine Source.

Actions & Effects of Geranium Essential Oil

Action Keywords; *Sense Of Safety, Internal Conflicts, Unite Soul Fragments, Broken Heart, Abandonment, Isolation, Shame, Divine Grace, Freedom Of Joyous Love*

Geranium brings the safety to confront issues that cause conflict, the energy transforming deep feelings and allowing for those fragmented aspects of Self to regroup and for a deeper bond with one's Soul energy to occur.

Resourcefulness is increased, the heart energy expands and a feeling of freedom leading to joy is possible.

The **Thymus** chakra is expanded, and unresolved past life memories can surface. These often depress the immune system, which can lead to negative feelings that include unworthiness, shame, injustice, abandonment and isolation.

Working on a **Soul** level, Geranium gently nurtures the emotional body to help heal rips and holes that have been caused by inharmonious emotions. Feelings of heartache, embarrassment and low self-esteem can diminish as the **Soul's** essence re-gathers its fragmented parts.

Vengeful or morbid thoughts or embarrassment can be addressed or cleared, as this works toward integration of one's shadow side. The magnetic energy that has locked these and other negative emotions in place can give way to trusting the flow of life again.

The **Thymus Chakra** which is connected to the Soul is greatly assisted with Geranium, as is the **Navel chakra, Third Eye** and Upper or **Higher Chakras**.

Meridians that are supported are the kidney, liver, bladder and the Central meridian.

More on Geranium Essential Oil

When used on the heart and breasts area, the oil feels very nurturing and stimulates greater self-acceptance.

Massage into the pineal gland points on the **Third Eye** area, the reflex points on the hands and feet for cellular regeneration.

It is often recommended for hormonal imbalances in females, but it also works on overall hormonal balance, including serotonin, dopamine, testosterone balance and many other hormones responsible for regulating and harmonizing the cycles and processes in the physical body.

<><><>

GRAPEFRUIT ESSENTIAL OIL

This is great Brain oil – that is it aids the brain to slow down the chatter, releasing and removing unwanted thoughtforms and allowing the mind to hear one's own inner thoughts. The control dial to the subconscious is turned down, and negative programming can be addressed.

Its scent is crisp and fresh, bringing the promise of lightness like a sparkling shower after heavy weather conditions.

It also brings a promise of the sun and light again.

Though it can be associated with food, it has hidden qualities and powers. As the humble grapefruit has the power to assist in clearing the palate with its distinctive aroma, when used in this concentrated form, its cleansing powers are quite amazing.

Etheric Colours of Grapefruit Essential Oil

Colour Codes; *Light and Dark Emerald Green, Violet, Yellow, Gold Flakes, Magenta*

The space that the bright Emerald Greens bring to the energy bodies will allow the mind to begin to clear and calm and peace is initiated. As the Greens travel through the auric systems it anchors this peace, engaging the heart. Violet then follows through to begin its energetic work.

This particular violet has a luminosity to it, and as the colour engages, it not only begins its transformation process, it also stimulates intuition, mysticism and inspiration as it acts to clear all the chakras, aligning them correctly with the **Crown Chakra**.

The Yellow then allows and attracts a stream from the Yellow spectrum. This works on bringing greater clarity to the mental body and more sunlight into the etheric fields.

Yellow gives way to Gold, initially as bubbles, which then become flakes that are attracted to and attach to where they are needed in the Light bodies.

A final wave of Magenta completes the process of Grapefruit, releasing residual grief and transporting more Divine Love into the being.

Actions & Effects of Grapefruit Essential Oil

Action Keywords; *Calm Mind Chatter, Inner Source Directives, Beliefs & Karmic Imprints, Fragmented Personality, Depression, Auric Density, Thoughtforms, Soul Purpose, New Realities, Core Energy, Mercury Retrograde*

Grapefruit oil aids the mental body to settle, and helps expand the **Heart** and **Third Eye** Chakras. The mental body calms and mind chatter settles.

Auric density caused by negative fall-out or toxic thoughts, no matter their original source, are cleared out, and the aura is able to recalibrate itself again.

It also soothes the **Solar Plexus Chakra**, aiding the personality to compose or recompose itself. This allows one's Core Energy to re-focus for ones' own inner source to make decisions and to create the new realities required for moving forward.

Depression is temporarily lifted to allow the release and replacement of the limiting thoughtforms that have perpetuated through the aura. The personality can now collect and reassert itself in a more positive light.

The **5ᵗʰ Earthing Chakra** in the New Earthing Chakra system is more easily accessed for better connection and grounding of the Major Chakra system. This creates a more comprehensive balance in the current climate of intense energy shifts.

Shock resonating within the etheric skeleton and accessed via the **Shoulder Chakras** (in the new **Signal Chakra system)** are also balanced as the combined energies of Magenta and Yellow create the Coral needed for this area.

The **Eye Chakras** are bathed with the luminous Violet and perceptions can be changed and harmonized as inner emotions are either released, transformed or regulated.

The doors to higher knowings can be accessed when worked with intentionally.

Meridians supported with Grapefruit are: kidney, stomach, lung and Governing.

More on Grapefruit Essential Oil

It is wonderful detoxification oil, great in a bath, or even a few drops added to body lotion to aid cellular and toxic release.

Use anytime to bring a lift or to remind yourself of the freshness that a new day can bring.

When Mercury is retrograde for three times every year for approximately three weeks, it can make communication difficult or throw up obstacles or cause us to go inward. Grapefruit can assist with assimilating the astrological energies and deal with the disruptions, lessening the confusions caused by it.

Secrets Beyond Aromatherapy

JASMINE ESSENTIAL OIL

The heady enveloping smell of Jasmine can remind one of a warm summer's evening and the sweetness of life again.

This gorgeous oil created from a hardy yet delicate and abundantly flowered plant, is often underestimated. Its ability to fill in holes in the aura is excellent. This provides a more comfortable place for the being, alleviating anxiety.

Often used in perfumes, this scent has a luxurious perfume to it, allowing the senses space to feel pleasure again.

Etheric Colours of Jasmine (Absolute) Essential Oil

Colour Codes; *Gold, Blue, Pink, Green, Violet, Silver*

Starting its etheric colour process with Gold and ending with Silver, this creates a comprehensive bath of supportive energies for all of the energy bodies.

A veritable rainbow of colour, one is hardly assimilated before the next follows on, overriding the senses to create a kind of bliss in the aura. Jasmine moves quickly but requires a little time for full effect.

As the Gold triggers Divine Source connection, the energy bodies are flooded with the Blue of calm and peace. We are signaled to release old emotions and sorrow. Pink then moves in to assist with balancing the heart and emotions to a higher vibration. The heart colour Green, for space and nurturing unlocks ones healing potential.

With this, we can glimpse better outcomes as Violet begins its transformation of negative to positive. Silver aligns us again to our personal power and we can again access our own power.

Actions & Effects of Jasmine Essential Oil

Action Keywords; *Good for Auric Holes, Protective, Self-Esteem, Tension, Anxiety, Confidence To Overcome Immediate Problems*

Gold is essential for auric health, which leads to etheric health. The aura is immediately boosted and auric holes begin to choose to knit again.

The protection from this oil allows us to address issues of alienation, separation and self-esteem that have created tension and anxiety.

Moving quickly through the aura, the **Heart Chakra** is activated, together with the senses. Our alignment to Source ensures the senses to be more aware of pleasure than our pain, giving one the space and confidence to overcome one's immediate problems.

Boosting the entire **Major Chakra** system, and strengthening not only our Core Energy but also our total Aura, the Crystalline Body is strengthened, and the auric layers align and harmonize.

Specific **Chakras** supported are **Heart, Thymus, Throat, Third Eye** and **Crown**.

Meridians that benefit are: lung, triple-warmer, spleen, bladder and Governing.

More on Jasmine Essential Oil

When working in groups or dealing with inharmonious family situations, this oil can help alleviate the pain experienced at the hands or actions of those we assume will love and accept us yet don't.

It is also excellent for psychic work and energy work due to its actions on the etheric body and its ability to repair the aura.

After a sudden shock, this is one of those supportive oils that give the space to heal again.

Precautions:

Always use diluted for topical skin application or massage, as with all of the other oils. Check on the purity of the oil as some times synthetics are used in inferior oil products.

TIPS

MORE STATEMENTS FOR **MERIDIANS**:

Lung Meridian:

> I am worthy
>
> I am tolerant
>
> I am modest

Kidney Meridian:

> I am courageous
>
> I am secure

Triple Warmer Meridian:

> I am at peace with myself
>
> I am relaxed

Juniper Essential Oil

Cleanses the emotional body to enable alignment to the Soul and Divine Source. Excellent for detoxification of the auric bodies.

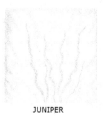

JUNIPER

Etheric Colours of Juniper Essential Oil

Colour Codes; *Silver Threads, White-Light, Blue*

The initial shiny threads of Silver produced by Juniper bathe the Soul body and ease nervous tension. Anxiety and shock is soothed, which allows easier access to the **Higher Chakras** above the head.

The oscillations produced through the frequency vibration of this oil can release stuck clouds of stagnant or poisoned energies which are then engulfed in the pure White that follows it.

This allows for one's personal Energy Ray and Colour Ray to bring nurturing and harmonious energies.

As the White-Light cleanses and purifies, it gives way to the Blue Light, which keys one back in to one's personal and inner truth. As this grounds one and connects into the **3rd Earthing Chakra** of one's innate humanity, this assists with a more peaceful alignment with one's ancestral chi, ancestral history and impetus, and eases existing conflict between one's DNA and Soul impulse.

Actions & Effects of Juniper Essential Oil

Action Keywords; *Patience, Soul Group Connection, Heart Alignment, Lost Faith, Feeling Love, Stagnant Energies, Pagan Lifetimes, Fairies & Elves*

Juniper Essential Oil is a powerful transition oil, assisting in promoting patience with not only the self, but also with one's own healing process. There is greater access to clean Chi.

As it clears toxic energies and brings alignment, a better connection toward one's **Source** and with one's **Soul** Group energies is experienced. This creates a greater sense of safety and assists with restoring lost faith.

As the **Heart Chakra** aligns with Divine Source, more spiritual love and self love can move back in.

Reminders of past lives where there was a more natural relation between one's spiritual life, and one's physical activities can take place. This assists in re-membering faith in the natural order of things, and in one's inner knowing, especially when living more connected with nature in pagan lifetimes.

For some, there can be a re-awakening of companionship with the unseen devic and nature realms of fairies and elves.

Juniper allows Protective Chi to filter through the auric bodies, and stimulates the Crystalline light structure of the etheric body as consciousness is stimulated.

Chakras supported are: 3rd **Earthing, Navel, Heart, Throat** and the **Third Eye**.

Meridians that benefit are: spleen, bladder and triple-warmer.

More on Juniper Essential Oil

Used as a room spray, it helps to eliminate toxic buildups and helps clear inharmonious emotions that have laden the atmosphere. Good after energy work or processes.

When a few drops are added to the bath, it assists in cleansing the aura of heavy emotions, so it is excellent when undergoing a detox or when wanting to soften buried or hardened emotions.

Precautions:

Do not use during pregnancy, or with children. Avoid direct skin contact without dilution.

Avoid using for longer than 3 months at a time, as it will build up in the system and may become toxic. Have periodic breaks of say 2 months in between continual applications of Juniper in any of its various forms.

TIPS

MORE STATEMENTS FOR **MERIDIANS**:

Gall Bladder Meridian:

> I can reach out with love
>
> I am being myself
>
> I am empowered
>
> I am in my own power

Large Intestine Meridian:

> I release the past, anger, worries and doubt safely
>
> I set new goals

Small Intestine Meridian:

> I appreciate myself
>
> I am satisfied

LAVENDER ESSENTIAL OIL

How could I not include the common Lavender? This profuse little plant can grow into a mighty bush, giving off its familiar perfume through its stems, leaves and flowers.

Lavender oil assists in aligning and expanding the Heart and Crown Chakra, particularly when they are in states of stress or fear. This allows a better flow of energy and brings balance and calmness to the being.

Lavender in the form of a Flower Essence is also useful for psychic protection & oversensitivity to psychic development or experiences.

Etheric Colours of Lavender

Colour Codes; *Silver-Gold, Blue-Green*

At first glance, it would appear there are only two colour codes, but these are actually a very potent and comprehensive combination.

The first emergence of the etheric colours is in the form of a spiral dance of Silver and Gold. Each of these etheric colours is separately very powerful, working on the etheric and subtle anatomy bodies and also on the Soul level. When they are combined together like this, they help soothe the Soul and strengthen the auric and subtle bodies to further hold the rebalanced energies. Silver assists with energetic communication, whilst Gold is essential to auric health. (A greater access to Divine Light is possible when the being begins to align.)

Blue-Green: We now allow for the combinations of not just Blue, and just Green, but the full spectrum range of each of these colours. Not only do we have all possible colours of Green, and all possible colours of Blue available to draw on but we also have all possible combinations of the turquoises and Teals. Chakra wise, this covers not only the heart and throat, but also our inner communication ability. This also means that the physical body can communicate its wants, needs and concerns and begin to find the appropriate inner resource to meet these.

Actions & Effects of Lavender

Action Keywords; *Eases Heartache, Reduces Tension and Stress, Enhances Sense of Security, Builds Self Trust, Grace, Allows Relaxation, Soothes Turmoil and Promotes Peace, Aids Sleep, Soothes Nervous System, Allows for New Intuitive Information*

On an etheric level, or when used during healing or balancing sessions, the action of Lavender can assist with supporting the revelation of past or painful issues through to an easier conclusion because of its action on the **Heart** and **Crown Chakra**.

Aligning the **Major Chakras** as it does brings greater peace, creating better communication with all aspects of the being again. The intensity of memories is reduced, which assists in feeling safer.

Chakras activated by this oil include **Heart**, **Throat** and **Crown**.

Meridians that benefit from Lavender include: Central, Governing and the lung meridian. Assisting with releasing grief, the emotions are thereby nurtured. For those who are sensitive, this can allow for a stronger sense of connection with guidance or the Angelic realm.

More on Lavender Essential Oil

Even though this oil has many widespread uses, it should never be underrated.

Its common uses in aromatherapy include: general overall balancing, aids sleep, protective, soothes the nervous system. It can be dabbed onto the temples to aid in stress Reduction.

Frequently used in the best wax furniture polish, Lavender is found in some form in most homes, either in the kitchen, bathroom or toilet. When used in Lavender furniture polish, the Lavender assists in removing negative emotional imprints that have attached to wood. Wood absorbs energetic explosions and powerful emotions over time, but this will help to clear energetically as well as enliven the surrounds and space.

Used in soaps, cleaning and disinfectant applications, hand creams, pomades and perfumes, and even in some tea caddies for a night time preparation.

Its antiseptic properties make it ideal for a room spray, whether spritzing up stale air, or to provide a calming and refreshing ambience in sick rooms, and even for clearing and steam cleaning carpets and mattresses.

A warm bath or footbath is a great way to prepare for sleep, working on many levels of a person; it provides soothing, helps clear toxins, calms the nervous system and eases the mind, especially when accompanied by a simple Lavender tea infusion. This can be made from your own little Lavender bush by simply infusing / soaking the leaves and flowers in hot water for a couple of minutes before sipping. For sleep you can also dab it directly onto the wrists in small amounts, and the temples just before retiring.

Sleeping Tip: Have your mattress professional cleaned by someone who uses Lavender oil in their process. Or make your own mattress spray with Lavender oil and turn regularly. It not only deters little bed visitors, it also clears energetic crap that has drained during sleep into the bed over time.

Insect bites and minor itches can be eased with straight Lavender oil. The raw lavender plant has even been used when the oil had run out; it was applied by rubbing the leaves and seeds on the bite, and a band-aid or sticking plaster held it in place for it to do its work. Fixed!

LEMON ESSENTIAL OIL

Lemon is useful to clear and focus the mind, and to make greater connections to one's inner joy and optimism. It assists with decisions and to clear confusions. It is an encouraging ray of sunshine.

Etheric Colours of Lemon Essential Oil

Colour Codes; *Green, Copper-Gold-ish Yellow, Slightly Violet*

Beginning with the Green of the heart center, it calms and prepares the being with the space for change from constriction.

The next vibration of Copper Gold Yellow is a direct ray of sunshine that brings clarity to the mental body whilst strengthening the energy fields and bringing the positive aspects of emotions. The Copper aspect supports the light bodies and lifts the mind.

Towards the end of the action, etheric codes of Violet show themselves within the Yellow. This brings about a spiritual connection, allowing one to gain spiritual support easily. This helps to guide better decision making, and to accept one's behaviors with more understanding.

Actions & Effects of Lemon Essential Oil

Action Keywords; *Inner Joy, Encourages Optimism, Ease Throat Chakra, Sharpens Mind, Alcohol Addiction Released From Cellular Memory, Cleansing, Cynicism, Scattered, Detoxification*

Access to further wisdom is achieved with Lemon Essential oil. The etheric colour and olfactory actions assist a sharper mind and cuts through confusions. Both calming and activating, Lemon brings more joy and optimism, and helps to cleans all energy bodies to lift the mood and bring a sense of hope.

Used in warm water and honey, it assists to ease stress in the throat, and aids clearer expression. It is great for cleansing the liver and gall bladder, and it can assist in the alcohol cleansing processes, as it helps to clear cellular memories of this and other potentially addictive substances.

It can also assist with cravings, particularly when massaged into the body.

The main Chakras that are supported are the **Sacral Chakra, Solar Plexus, Heart Chakra, Throat Chakra** and the **Ear Chakras.**

Meridians and organs that benefit from Lemon are: Liver, gall bladder, kidneys and the stomach.

More on Lemon Essential Oil

Lemon used daily assists in eliminating stress from the mind & aura. Used as a spray, it is good for psychic self protection, and also for clearing stale or emotionally charged energy in any space.

It can be used to cheer up hospital 'inmates' as well as help clear the space.

LEMONGRASS ESSENTIAL OIL

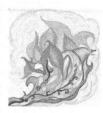

LEMONGRASS

A highly spiritual essential oil, this interesting and uniquely perfumed oil is a tonic to the etheric body and aura. Often used to combat stress from electromagnetic and electrical bombardment, it is great for those working around computers and electrical equipment.

Etheric Colours of Lemongrass

Colour Codes; *Purple, Red, Orange, Green*

The first colour code and action is Purple – bright, vivid and rich - stimulating the **Crown Chakra**, energetically invigorating the brain, and working to strengthen the aura and its own electromagnetic properties. Having activated the **Crown Chakra** we move into:

Red: This activates our vitality potential, and assists with grounding. As the anatomy engages we can initiate action on some level of our being. With a clearer outlook through the Purple, 'rat race' tendencies are diminished, and through the Red our life force energy is activated. Yellow now enters the colour code equation and so we move into:

Orange: The emotional body is now balanced and realigned. This assists in soothing the mental body. There is more joy and lightness available now.

Finally Green brings us further up the Major Chakra system and into a sense of nurturing as the energy stimulates and activates us back into one's heart space as the **Heart Chakra** is supported.

The overall effect is this... Firstly there is a clearing of negative energies, and a 'calling-in' on the spiritual level to enlist one's spiritual or inner forces. The Red then provides and activates grounding energies, and confers vitalization to move forward on both a physical level and on an energetic level. As this is then followed by Orange, it indicates the rebalancing on an emotional level, also assisting with the release of emotions that may have been held due to shock or crisis. The Green allows the space and nurturing to process these emotions (and shock resonances) without the need to re-experience them again unnecessarily.

As Green is also the heart colour, this works to place us back in our heart again, and to bring us back to the present moment in time and space.

Actions & Effects of Lemongrass

Action Keywords; *Electro-Magnetic Field Shield, Purifies Etheric, Repairs Auric Holes, Rat Race & Pressure, Pesky Irritations, Optimism, Courage to Overcome, Nervous System Calmed, Future Fears Eased*

Like a breath of fresh spring air, Lemongrass uplifts the mind and body. The **Heart Chakra** is strengthened, the **Base Chakra** is supported, and the **Sacral Chakra** is soothed and eased.

The Aura is greatly enhanced. The nervous System, particularly along or up the spine, is 'washed' and re-invigorated.

Residual memories or imprints of a recent nature can be sloughed off. It can also assist with parasitic energies, particularly caused by denied emotion infections from others. Like Citronella, it is useful for supporting the nervous system and cleaning up from tiny energetic invaders.

Chakras that are positively impacted are: **Heart Chakra, Base Chakra, Throat Chakra and the Crown Chakra.**

Use to cleanse and strengthen the astral body, etheric body and the emotional body.

Meridians that benefit include: gall bladder, spleen, large intestine and central meridians.

More on Lemongrass

Pessimism can be eased using Lemongrass Essential Oil, and more positive options and a healthier outlook open up in challenging situations. The brain can open new pathways, and clearer thinking can be generated.

'Wiping' the aura near the **Solar Plexus** and **Sacral Chakras** can clear buildup of toxic fog. Electromagnetic fug (a kind of energetic 'phlegm' that can clog up energy flow) is cleared from the etheric body, and the aura can be recover to repair itself and allow for further energetic enhancement.

Add to your bath to absorb more vitalizing energy into the etheric and auric fields.

<><><>

TIPS

MORE STATEMENTS FOR **MERIDIANS**:

Circulation-Sex Meridian:

> I forgive the judgements I have placed against myself

> I forgive the judgements others have placed against me

Stomach Meridian:

> I nurture myself with good things

> I take care of my own business

Liver Meridian:

> I take responsibility for myself and my actions

> I do not take responsibility for the actions of others

> I am happy and cheerful

LEMON MYRTLE ESSENTIAL OIL

Lemon Myrtle tends to release a song of etheric colours that activates as they are released. Like the 'notes' of perfume from this tune of vibrational energy, each brings a differing action into play.

So you can expect the healing energy of the etheric action of Lemon Myrtle to initially start her colour palette with a 'chord of Green.

Lemon Myrtle Etheric Properties and Action

Colour Codes; *Spectrum Green, Gold, Pink*

Spectrum Green **b**rings all of the different hues and shades of Green into play. From Olive Green to Lime Green, from Emerald Green, Verdant Green, to Spring Green and Chartreuse. Each shade or hue of Green is only absorbed as it is required or needed.

Green provides a clearing, a space that is neutral and supportive. Each Green has its own unique action, and so when using spectrum Green, we are combining the many beneficial aspects of the different ranges of Green that vary from inner leadership, to physical nurturing, and nurturing of the emotional aspects in present time.

Next, Lemon Myrtle brings the action and note together with the etheric colour of Yellow **Gold**. As the Spectrum Green has a nurturing yet space-giving effect on the energy systems of the body, this is an ideal space to then bring in the **Auric** strengthening properties of Gold.

This then allows for more assimilation of the **Energy of Light**.

We often get caught up with the 'shades' of life, and get a bit blocked in our ability to process the light that is all around us. It doesn't have to be the sunlight, just any daylight. If we work or stay in fluorescent lights a lot, we can have an imbalance from lack of the full spectrum of light which can feel like and create a 'draining' effect on our energy and energy systems, particularly for sensitive types.

Next we move onto Pink – Palest Pink of a slightly Violet hue through to a warm middle Pink, tending to be of the gentler, warmer, almost spiritual hues, rather than the vibrant hot Pink hues.

As you will most probably know, Pink has been the new **Heart Chakra** colour for some time, as it brings in a spiritual energy. Pink (like Green) is a heart center balancing colour, and is also seen as the colour of love. So the result of the actions of Spectrum Green then Gold, then Pink combines to calm, strengthen and then balance, which allows the **Chakra** systems to reset again, and the heart to renew.

Actions & Effects of Lemon Myrtle

Action Keywords; *Electro-Magnetic Fields, Light Assimilation & Aura Balancing, Male / Female Inner Balance, Resolve Internal Conflicts, Sumerian Past Lives, Past Life Secrets of Form & Nature*

Starting off as it does with the full spectrum of Green, we immediately move into heart space. The strengthening provided by the Gold begins to support or re-build our personal electromagnetic field.

Coming from this heart space and embracing the more spiritual Pinks, we can access and resolve certain memories and gifts.

Past live experiences as being male or female are addressed or revealed, which can allow for better access to the original imbalances in order to achieve greater integration and balance in this gender life choice. Because of this action-ability, the oil can resurrection past issues for resolution or simply empower us to access the gifts of both strengths and qualities.

Lemon Myrtle enhances the **Base Chakra, Sacral Chakra, Heart Chakra, Crown Chakra** and the **Higher Chakras.**

Meridians that gain great benefit from Lemon Myrtle are Governing, liver, kidney and gall bladder.

The astral body is cleansed and strengthened. It is recharged and this further supports the mental body. The etheric body is settled and soothed allowing for greater co-operation in all energy fields. The aura can expand in a stronger, more defined and cohesive way.

Electro-Magnetic Fields

Like Lemongrass, this is a great oil for being around devices that can affect our electromagnetics, such as electrical equipment, computers, wireless gadgets or equipment that use or can conduct, transmit, broadcast or diffuse electrical or magnetic spectrum waves.

You can make a simple spray and use it in your aura to 'spritz' and enliven the normal electro-magnetics again, or use around computer stations to clear the air or space from positive or charged ions.

Light Assimilation & Aura Balancing

There are other levels of use for this beautiful oil. Besides assisting with Light Assimilation (important at this time of planetary changes), it can also assist with our connecting and merging to our **Spiritual** nature with ease. This brings more balance and light into the **Aura**. (A great way to enhance the energy fields, energy store and total aura.)

Lemon Myrtle assists also with the assimilation of the higher vibrations of light. This brings a greater appreciation and understanding of the nature of merging into oneness and also of being truly individual.

To best use this oil's colour codes, be aware of Conscious *Directed* breathing it deeply not just into your electrical systems in the brain, nervous systems and body, but also into your **Chakras** and / or meridians (if you are aware of them) and into your **Aura** to reset your electro-magnetic fields. This friendly oil really wants to help balance you and bring you back into more of a sense of oneness with yourself again. Right now, with all of the challenges that many are facing, this is particularly helpful.

More on Lemon Myrtle

Certain Past Life memories can be stimulated together with their gifts. Such as ancient Sumerian lives or connections with the Goddess Aphrodite and Marienna ('Mother of Heaven'), as well as skills in wisdom and consciousness regarding the forms of nature and matter, and the cycling of life.

Applying to the base of the skull and **4 ½ Chakra** or **Zeal Point Chakra** helps to align the body templates for greater energy flow and assimilation, and greater ability to be more in the present moment.

This oil can also assist a sluggish pituitary gland; firmly massage and press the centre of the big toe which is the reflex point, while inhaling deeply.

LIME ESSENTIAL OIL

Lime Essential Oil helps ease trauma in the cellular memory. It also is excellent for cleansing and revitalizing the energy bodies.

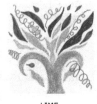

LIME

Use it to remind you of the potential playfulness and innocence of the child within.

Etheric Colours of Lime Essential Oil

Colour Codes; *Green, Gold, Blue, Magenta*

Its initial effect of Green, is similar to the Lemon Essential oil. Moving directly into Gold, the whole of the energy bodies are not only strengthened, but there is a sense of real support and connection back to the 'brighter' side of life'

Gold works on all levels of the being, helping one to connect back to one's Source. The etheric effects move through the light bodies and leave a film of sheen and brightness, as the sequence moves into Blue.

Blue brings with it one's inner truth and knowing, one's own codes. This assists with self recognition and protection. Blue after Gold also helps set the tone of the electromagnetic field, cleansing and re-aligning it.

The final tone is the flow of Magenta, which helps with aligning to spiritual aspects of physical life. It is supportive, nurturing, and caring.

Actions & Effects of Lime Essential Oil

Action Keywords; *Cellular Memory Soothed, Cleanse, Joy, Revitalize, Trauma, Etheric Salve, Lightness, Laughter, Inner Child & Body Issues, Cord Cutting, Karmic*

Working on many levels and bodies, Lime Essential oil assists with the child within. Frozen memories that have been stuck in time, or kept us stuck in time, and that are emerging can be eased and moved on with this uplifting oil. The energy bodies especially the Astral and Soul light bodies, are relieved of their energy burdens from others, particularly in the form of ties or cords.

Energy drains leading to others can be disconnected and this oil is great for use in any form of energy cutting ceremony, meditation or process. For Karmic cords connecting us to others or to other places or things, using Lime oil will assist in the clearing process.

Fear or heavy density in the etheric light bodies holding one back, will be alleviated and disconnected.

This oil reminds us of love and joy again. It also works on etheric scars and traumatic wounds, and is a salve to the whole body. Lime helps the energy of the Soul to come through again.

The chakras it focuses on are: **Navel Chakra, Heart Chakra, Throat Chakra** and the **Hand Chakras.** Working on these chakras allows more light of Soul and Self, and more willingness to receive again, this time in safety.

Lime Essential oil works on: the Etheric body, physical body, mental body, **Soul body** and the **Astral body.**

The Meridians that benefit from focus or massage are: the Central and Governing meridians, heart, lung, kidney and gall bladder meridians.

More on Lime Essential Oil

You can use this delightful oil on any area of the body that holds unhappy memories, or cellular trauma: operations, broken bones, physical attacks, anchored experiences. For instance - When someone has been forced to do something they didn't want to do, and the body was held (down, back, tied up, chained etc), it can create an 'anchor' for the memory in the body.

Such as one small boy who was held by his wrists to be forced to have lots of necessary but very painful injections. His wrists held the traumatic memories as an anchor, and when unwary teachers later went to get hold of him by his wrists, he relived the memory and became quite uncontrollable and wild.

Lime adds well with other oils that are heavy, to bring a lift to the process and experience. It works well with Nutmeg Essential oil for issues of betrayal.

TIPS

MORE STATEMENTS FOR **MERIDIANS**:

Spleen Meridian-

> I have confidence in my future
>
> I am secure
>
> I trust myself

Bladder Meridian:

> I am confident about my future
>
> I manage my desires and release yearnings
>
> I am at peace

General Meridian Statement:

> I have love, faith, trust, gratitude and courage

NUTMEG ESSENTIAL OIL

Using Nutmeg Essential oil will help with easing attachment issues, and bringing a sense of liberation around issues and people connected with betrayal and loss.

It helps bring some light and ease the pain when one feels in a 'black hole' of dark emotion.

Etheric Colours of Nutmeg Essential Oil

Colour Codes;   *Red, Orange, Yellow, Blue With Green Tinge, Purple*

Initiating action with the Red colour code, life force is encouraged to enliven the aura, bringing an action energy that is also very protective.

This allows for the energy to address issues of emotions, as we move into the Orange mode. Orange is a great colour to settle shock. It also reminds us of the possibility of joy, whilst helping to re-balance those emotions that are not in balance. All emotions are appropriate, but when we are stuck in an emotion, it creates an imbalanced tone and emotion which affects the flow of energy.

Yellow brings clarity and assists with settling the mental body. Yellow is commonly associated with sunshine, and sand, and freedom, and so it is here. As the Yellow creates its gentle pulse through the etheric, Limitations begin to easy, and we continue up the chakra system to the throat area.

Blue-Green: Blue of the throat supports our ability to hold strong in the face of truth. When tinged with the Green, this brings the heart into play, to assist with healing the rigidity experienced in the body, heart and psyche.

The final frequency of Purple surrounds the light bodies and ensures transmutation and transformation on all levels. It also brings us full circle with the Major Chakra system, starting from the Base chakra and ending with the Crown chakra.

Actions & Effects of Nutmeg Essential Oil

Action Keywords; *Betrayal & Loss Eased, Spontaneity, Flexibility, Detachment, Rigidity, New Foundations, Heart Dance with Joy, Wild & Free*

The power of Nutmeg moves the pain and hurt in the heart in the cases of loss or betrayal in a relationship. It shatters illusions to reveal the truth, which allows for closure. Detachment is enabled. Rejection is eased. We begin to find ourself again.

When we have become too serious, or we are in danger of sliding into darkness, pessimism or hopelessness, Nutmeg will help to arrest this and will ease more light into our future.

Loss of sentimental items can be eased with Nutmeg. Our ability to establish new future foundations is encouraged as the bands around our heart are eased and loosened.

We learn to dance with joy again, and to remember the feel of freedom.

The total **Major Chakra system** is supported with Nutmeg Essential Oil. The new evolved Human Earthing Chakras that are enhanced and assisted in better balance are: **3rd, 4th, 5th**, and the **8th Earthing Chakras**.

Meridians that are well supported with Nutmeg are: the Governing meridian (backache and the spine is eased in cases of feeling lack of support), spleen and liver.

The emotional body is soothed, the astral body is eased, the Soul body is supported and the aura reactivates itself to a higher level of protective and supporting function.

More on Nutmeg Essential Oil

Good for lower back pain, digestive problems, and assisting with activation in the morning. As it is invigorating in its energy action, do not use too late in the day as it may prevent quick sleep.

This is a power oil and when used in large quantities, may be hallucinogenic, so limit its use.

Precautions:

Do not use on children. Avoid during pregnancy. Do not overuse in case of headaches. Dilute 1-10 drops in 2 ounces of base oil before topical application on the skin. Limit to 1-5 drops when used in a bath.

Secrets Beyond Aromatherapy

ORANGE (SWEET) ESSENTIAL OIL

Orange Essential Oil brings a sweetness and a lift from the first breathe. We can feel the benefits begin quickly. It brings promise of lightness with it.

Etheric Colours of Orange Essential Oil

Colour Codes; *Purple, Silver Light, Gold, White*

Depending on the particular quality of the Essential Oil, you can expect the following etheric and colour vibrations from the Orange family, and in particular from Sweet Orange.

One would expect that the essential oil of Orange would be the same colour: that of Orange. But instead, it starts off with the almost the opposite on the colour wheel.

The initial release of vibrational healing colour is Purple. This is generally followed by Silver light, then Gold.

The effect is quite strengthening on the aura overall.

Finally, the White Ray shines through, assisting with overall balance.

The sequencing is this: The appearance of the initial colour code of Purple in the energy field assists with the transformation or transmutation of negative energies of all kinds. This means that any negative energy caught up in one's energy field begins to dissipate and alter into more friendly useable energy. If we could liken its cleansing action to common kitchen cleansers, then this acts more as a gentle yet powerful cleanser (and where necessary, a gentle sparkly polish) rather than bleach on a scourer.

The colour code of Silver Light assists with flexibility, ease of communication and assists in harmonizing emotions with expression. Silver Light also supports the **Soul** aspects, and assists with Soul related issues.

Moving to Gold, creates a strengthening and 'seal'-ing effect, which holds the benefits and protects them like flexible armor, particular when experienced immediately after the Silver-Light.

Actions & Effects of Orange Essential Oil

Action Keywords; *Purifies Emotional and Astral Body, Auric Density Eased, Repels Negative Entities, Judgmentalism, Drama, Obsession*

The powerful affect from such a common and easily accessible oil and food is quite interesting. It has a reputation for lightening the emotions, allowing space for more positive emotions in our life, such as joy.

On an energetic level, we can see more clearly how this is done, and how it impacts on the energy bodies and brain.

It initially works on balancing and cleansing the density in the **Aura** and **Astral** bodies, so that strong emotions are calmed, entities are repelled and the aura begins to clear.

Helping to break through the intensities accumulated in the energy fields of fears, drama, or over-judgmental-ism, this essence further works on the aura and assists it to begin to repair itself. This will enhance and support your energy fields, your energy reserves and strengthen the aura.

Obsessions can begin to recede and rectify themselves. Leaches such as minor entities are loosened, imprints detach, elementals Redeploy.

It is easier to access **Spiritual** Subtle Bodies and centering becomes possible again.

Chakras that are activated or affected by Orange oil are: the **Link Chakra, Sacral Chakra, Heart Chakra, Crown Chakra** and the **Higher Self** *or* **I Am Chakra.**

Meridians that are supported and enhanced with Orange are – liver, lung, small intestine, heart and the Governing meridian.

More Information on Orange Essential Oil

It can be used to assist in repair of the energy fields after a shock as this can leave the aura 'battered' and open to invading energies. To do this, mix with a carrier oil, and it can then be rubbed on the left side of the body, particularly around the spleen area which is located on the inside of the left ribs. Use this mixture in an up and down movement to assist in sealing the energy fields and to prevent the escape of one's own energy.

The colour Orange, which is the colour of the host fruit of this essential oil, is renowned for its positive effects on the Emotional Body and when treating energetic displacement. Even though there is no Orange colour in Sweet Orange, because of its origin, it is excellent for after treating shock, trauma or drama. It is also helpful when having been exposed to drug users, particularly who one is closely connected with, such as friends or family.

Direct use of Orange oil can be slightly irritating. Don't expose the skin directly to the sun after use of this oil.

Take care when using on children.

Ensure good quality or organic oil if using directly on skin. Orange oil of a lesser quality is also useful for cleaning solid surfaces such as laminates or tiles, particularly on stubborn sticky or greasy areas, but can be drying to the hands.

<><><>

Secrets Beyond Aromatherapy

PALMAROSA ESSENTIAL OIL

Energy of Mother Earth. Manifestation and creation energies. Healing mother-child issues. Relationship matters.

Etheric Colours of Palmarosa Essential Oil

Colour Codes; *Magenta, Green, Dark Yellow, Pinkish*

Magenta is often used for those who care for others, and to remind us to enjoy the details or little things in life. When Magenta embraces us with her magic etheric codes, she reminds us that we are in a physical body which naturally houses spiritual love. This supports us with spiritual energy and earth energy again.

Moving into the Green of Palmarosa, we find our hearts responding, as space is made to examine the disparities that have led us away from balance in our lives and hearts.

As the Green moves to a transparent version, it gives way to Dark Yellow. Almost an olive green but not quite, it nevertheless strengthens the inner female in her positive traits, allowing for self mothering and nurturing. This alleviates self (and other) restrictions, allowing more freedom to create and birth new ideas, friendships, relationships, projects and wonder in life.

Ending with the pinkish codes, we bring gentleness back into the equation.

Pink softens the harshness of the base and sexual areas, areas connected on a deep level with birth, life and death, and with the instigation of life, so that conception and gestation memories and imprints that are painful or bring us anger can be dealt with in a way that nurtures us.

Actions & Effects of Palmarosa Essential Oil

Action Keywords; *Divine Mother Energy, Love & Compassionate Acceptance, Role Models, Need To Be 'Perfect', Childhood, Abandonment*

Whilst providing support to our energy systems, Palmarosa calls us to attention in the little things in our everyday life. Attention to mindfulness reconnects us back to ourselves again, which opens us up to better role models and innate understandings of our ability to mother ourselves. We may often forget this, but this oil assists us with her Magenta first energy. As magenta has the ability to connect us via the heart, its energy is also akin to Grace.

With intent, we can utilize the hidden potentials of this oil to self-parent and open to nurturing.

Childhood issues can be moved through more easily if there was hurt, shame, blame or pain. It is also useful when faced with child and parent matters, such as bonding, linking, mother-blame and love/hate issues.

Incarnational issues over choice of or treatment by parents can be more easily resolved and assimilated, as this oil can work on the following chakras: **Soul Star Chakra, Heart Chakra, Link Chakra.** These chakras play prime roles on the soul's path, so are greatly assisted to yield up their issues for healing.

Meridians that can be assisted with Palmarosa are: stomach, Central, heart and large intestine.

The mental body, astral body and causal light body are assisted with the etheric actions and colours.

This allows for easier relationships, and the ability to refocus our energies for the purposes of manifesting our creations in a loving way.

More on Palmarosa Essential Oil

When Palmarosa is in medicinal approved form, it can be taken orally (take care over dosages) for intestinal bacteria and Candida Albicans overgrowth.

It can also be helpful for nervous exhaustion if of a good quality. Blending with Lavender, Cedarwood and YlangYlang produces a fragrant and supportive mixture to calm and soothe the nervous system.

TIPS

STATEMENTS FOR **CHAKRAS**:

General Chakras:

I am receptive and responsive

Crown Chakra:

I am on purpose.

I have direction

Base Chakra:

I know what I want

It is safe to 'have', without harm to myself or others

My life force is in balance

Navel Chakra:

I am connected to myself

Patchouli Essential Oil

Reconnecting to the will to live and to open again to the nurturing forces of nature are just some of the gifts of Patchouli oil. The 'Blues' are addressed and survival fears are assisted with a renewal or increase of faith.

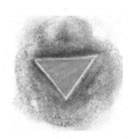

PATCHOULI

Also helpful when over-meditating and after intensive visualization or spiritual exercises to bring one back into the body again.

The aura is expanded and nurtured, as well as grounded. This helps in protecting the psyche.

Etheric Colours of Patchouli Essential Oil

Colour Codes; *Red/Orange, Violet tinged with Purple-Gold*

As the power of Red supports the life force energies it also stimulates the **Base Chakra**, the **Sacral Chakra** and **Sex Chakras**, as they are bathed in the Red and Orange and thus nurtured toward the rebuilding of vitality again. The Base or Root Chakra is opened, allowing for the grounding of the energy bodies and the nurturing of nature to aid in any spiritual endeavor or experience.

Emotions are balanced, and as the Violet begins to form, one is aligned to Soul energy, and beliefs and emotions are open to transformation and cleansing.

The Violet now forms Purple edges, with hints of Gold.

The Purple ignites one's spirituality and connection to Divine Source, whilst the Gold supports our wisdom and strengthens all bodies, aura and chakras. These Golden edges plume out further as they recede into the ethers, giving the appearance of a golden crown atop a reddish bulb.

Actions & Effects of Patchouli Essential Oil

Action Keywords; Grounding, Will To Live, Growth/Change, Survival, Sexual Issues, Value Life, The 'Blues', Suicidal, Intimacy, Sensuality

Overall, this oil grounds and activates the physical body whilst giving a sense of respect and value for life. The 'Blues' and suicidal tendencies can be eased, and one opens to the possibility of the life spark within each being. The physical form of our being is willing to feel more joy again, and to accept the responsibilities of living with the desire to change and grow.

Sexual issues, intimacy and the senses are addressed. Consciousness is expanded to allow for change and to revere the senses rather than to abuse them. The mental and etheric bodies are revived, and we view life in a more protective way. Patchouli oil is excellent for working with the **Earthing Chakras**.

It also benefits and balances the **Heart Chakra** and grounds the **Third Eye Chakra**. The pressure within the **Throat Chakra**, relaxes easing and freeing one's ability to express wants or needs.

Use during massage on the following meridians for improved functionality and to nourish: Central and Governing, Lung, Spleen, Large Intestine, Gall Bladder, Kidney and Bladder. The astral body is reordered and redefined and the mental body is recharged.

More on Patchouli Essential Oil

Massage in a base oil into the **Base Chakra** and **Sacral Chakra** to help clear and heal suicidal thoughts, as well as along the soles of the feet to aid grounding.

Chakras: **Base, Sacral, Heart, Third Eye, Throat,** and **Earthing Chakras**. Meridian and trunk massage allows joy to enter again.

PEPPERMINT ESSENTIAL OIL

When I was first introduced to this essential oil as an etheric colour code, with its association with confectionery, chewing gum and toothpaste etc I was not prepared for what I discovered.

Its ability to increase **Spiritual** energy and unblock physical energy is usually not as speedily or commonly recognized as its association with its 'crisp'ness energy. Metaphysically it assists with balancing the **Mental** body and calming its fears and mind chatter.

Etheric Colours of Peppermint

Colour Codes; *Pinks & Greens, Metallic Blue, Silvery Light*

Pinks & Greens: The heart colour codes of Green spectrum are further strengthened on a **High Heart Chakra** level with the Pink spectrum.   This creates a balance of the Twin Hearts, allowing for expansion in the heart of love and acceptance.   This flows through into:

Metallic Blue: The Blue colour code now allows movement up to the throat, and in this metallic form, it resonates on a higher vibration.   As a major connection point to the **Soul** body resides between heart and throat zones, the Soul is touched and influenced, balanced and infused. The **Mind** is able to settle.

Silvery Light: The Silver frequency further supports inner communication at a **Soul** level, allowing for higher truths to be accessed – not necessarily by the conscious mind, but by the aura and energy bodies, for the purpose of rebuilding the geometric aspects of the energy body Blueprints.

Actions & Effects of Peppermint

Action Keywords;   *Sacred Symbols & Geometry, Soul Truths, Higher Mind, For Terror, Hysteria, Fear of*

Unknown, Mind Chatter, Grounds 3rd Eye, Stomach, Resistance, Night Sweats

The previous section explains a lot of the action of Peppermint. However, for better understanding, here are further benefits and effects from it.

If there is some resistance within the body on an energetic level, this oil works on the **Etheric** to allow better energy flow within the body that can cause possible pain in the legs, or even migraine due to incompatibility of spiritual and physical energy. Peppermint helps to facilitate a better flow between the two.

When there is on an internal level some fear, terror or resistance, the geometric and symbolic building blocks of creation and matter are facilitated and translated to assist the light body to expand. Besides using the *Direct Inhalation* technique, apply Peppermint to the Crown and the soles of the feet and visualize the etheric colours and energies running up and down the body for a few times to assist with breaking up any resistance.

The **Third Eye Chakr**a aligns with the central nervous system stem along the spine, and grounds spirituality into the physical at the **Base chakra**. Through this action, the central Chakra core stem held in the spine allows for connection along the total **Main** or **Major Chakra system**, though the main effects are demonstrated through the Base and Third Eye. **Minor Chakras** at the joints are positively supported.

Therefore the Chakras activated by Peppermint Essential oil are: Base, Third Eye, and High Heart

Meridians that benefit from Peppermint oil action are the spleen, gall bladder, Governing and the bladder.

The Cerebral Cortex is enhanced for greater thought clarity. This allows easier access to the higher mind as the brain is supported for higher processes and access to higher levels of thinking.

More on Peppermint Essential Oil

The metaphysical properties of Peppermint essential oil also assist with the digestion and processing of new thoughts and beliefs on a mind level. Though the Peppermint tea is a greatly diluted form of the oil, it still creates a resonance that assists in settling the stomach. This is an echo on the physical level reflecting the metaphysical benefits.

It is not recommended to use too close to sleep unless it is a hot night, in which case it is best diluted with a carrier oil or body lotion so that it can be rubbed on the body for its cooling action.

Esoterically it has been linked with the god Horus, who was known for protection and wisdom. (For the cosmically minded, it has also been associated with Griffins.)

Note: Peppermint oil may reduce the effectiveness of homeopathic remedies. Do not apply neat when massaging the total body.

PETITGRAIN ESSENTIAL OIL

Power struggles, internal conflicts, integration of the self, and auric damage are all assisted with Petitgrain essential oil. Good for Grounding.

Etheric Colours of Petitgrain Essential Oil

Colour Codes; *Greenish-Yellow with Golden Sheen, Copper-Orange*

The unusual Greenish-Yellow theme of Petitgrain is an interesting colour code. It is more an intermingling of the two colours rather than a blending, which would have produced an Olive Green. Instead, two separate colour code actions combine to link together the green of the heart area and the yellow of the solar plexus.

However, it also works on settling an over-energized base chakra system, bringing the possibility of connecting to an easier sense of space and injecting the fresh-decision-making ability of the green into any turmoil, anger or frozen anguish that may be held in the solar plexus or base chakra systems.

As yellow is always a good colour code for the mental body, the actions combine to bring more 'sunshine' or golden-light energy into the energy fields. Gold supports the energy fields, and the aura is immediately supplied with the raw materials to begin rebuilding any damage from rigidity held in the meridian and chakra systems.

Turning to a Copper-Orange, the aura further benefits from the extra electrical conductivity of Copper, whilst also receiving the burst of bio-electric support into the etheric body that the Orange brings. This effective combination also assists with issues that have any 'shock' or trauma history or effect, and supports the being to repair any etheric damage.

Actions & Effects of Petitgrain Essential Oil

Action Keywords; *Overcome Obsessions & Addictions, Power Struggles, Internal Conflicts, Self Love, Acceptance, Anguish, Shame, Auric Rips, Heart Energy*

When feelings have become frozen, and in some cases, 'numb', this oil can assist to nurture us back to a willingness to embrace life again. Pain is enhanced when we have damaged energy systems, and this oil can assist with healing and rebuilding these again. This can allow us to engage again without unrealistic fears, or disproportionate or imagined pain.

The heart is supported, and negative mind talk can be eased. The back of the heart is where we often bury stuff 'back there' that we don't want to know about, don't want to feel, don't know how to deal with, or are so painful that we want to hide them or run away. When it is supported like this, we can begin to break old patterns. This oil can also assist with breaking habits.

Chakras: The main chakras that are engaged with this oil are: the **Sacral Chakra, Solar Plexus Chakra**, the **back of the Heart Chakra**. Though the action is not directly on the **Base Chakra**, it shifts an over energized Base Chakra to a more free flowing state, and assists with freeing up frozen conditions held within the energy bodies.

Use on the following meridians for enhanced energy and functionality: liver, heart, lungs, kidneys, gall bladder and large intestine.

The Etheric light body, emotional body, astral body, and the electromagnetic body all gain benefit from using Petitgrain. The coppery sheen in the etheric-action allows for better internal communication, co-operation and coordination of the energy systems.

More on Petitgrain Essential Oil

It has a reputation for assisting with convalescing and recovery from illness, as well as nervous exhaustion. It has also been used in cases of anxiety, and is a good anti-depressant. As it is excellent for rebuilding auric fields, it allows for awareness and acceptance, instead of harsh judgments or addictions.

ROSE OTTO ESSENTIAL OIL

Pure full strength Rose oil can often be quite expensive. It is excellent for energetic protection as it strengthens the aura, and is excellent for heartbreak, depression and grief. It is a very versatile all-rounder.

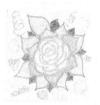

ROSE OTTO

The colour codes of Rose can be hard to pin down, due to the amazing variety of Roses and the vibrational codes which are affected by their land of origin and their cultivation environment. Not only can the colours of their blooms be affected but also the degree of perfume. Each colour also gives a different code and frequency, but though generally the Rose Otto uses a variety of coloured petals they are usually similarly perfumed and related in frequency ranges.

With this in mind the colour code reading provided here is for the Rose Otto that is most commonly used for essential oils and aromatherapy. This is a good basic guide, and if you sense or intuit that other colours come into your awareness when you use your essential oil, then this is obviously related to the individuality of the rose and the brand used and is absolutely fine.

Etheric Colours of Rose Otto

Colour Codes; *Roman Pink, Teal Green, Blue Spectrum, Gold & Silver*

Rose allows for the rainbow energies of Light to be accessed, bathing the energy bodies in healing and soothing rays. The interesting thing is that not all rainbow colours are seen etherically, though the affect on the aura would appear to be a full rainbow bath.

Following the colour codes generally and most often seen etherically the general indications of these usual etheric colours occur in this way:

164

Roman Pink can be described as a rich blush Pink, not as bright and vibrant as a full on flirty-Pink, but an intense hue of a gentle Pink. Sounds a bit contradictory? Well, the colour is just that – it is gentle, yet it is intense. This particular pink also settles energetic eruptions.

Pink is the new upgrade of the heart center, Green being the original **Heart Chakra** colour, but with the dawning and reclaiming of the 'High Heart' and the joining of the **'Twin Hearts'** within each of us, Pink is here to stay. Pink is the combination of Red and all of its qualities, together with White-Light, which brings it up to a higher spectrum of frequencies, utilizing and incorporating all of the qualities of both the Red and pure White-Light. This brings spirituality and grounding together in the heart space.

When this is followed by Teal Green, you bring in a greater ability for the heart and throat to connect. Teal assists this re-connection between the **Heart** and **Throat Chakras**, and also strengthens the ability for better self expression or self understanding.

Chakra wise, this lovely oil works not only with the Heart and Throat, but also our inner communication ability with all of the Main or Major **Chakras**. It also allows for **Soul** re-connection.

Actions & Effects of Rose Otto

Action Keywords; *Rainbow of Humanity, Unconditional Love, Relationships, Divine Stewardship, Transmute Burdens, Trust, Self Love, Soul Creativity, Inner Peace*

The spiraling centers of the rose can resemble a chakra, and rose assists the chakras to open correctly. The petals show gentleness and softness, yet they are often protected by thorns. Rose assists in breaking down defensiveness represented by these thorns to allow the energy of Spirit provide protection.

Rose is the rainbow after rain. It represents the **Spirit** and love.

Rose Otto Essential Oil is very powerful, and a **Heart** opener. As it begins its work in this way, all of the things shutting one down begin to surface.

Rose seems to reflect the complexity and evolution of life on Earth, not just for plants but also in their continually evolving ability to support humanity. It is a true 'Empress' amongst flowers and their essences in any form.

It is excellent for relationships, and brings in love in real and realistic way. Clingy-ness, jealousy and low self-esteem can be addressed. The action keywords listed pretty much describe its possibilities and applications.

Rose opens us to peace and assists transmuting what it is to be human. When it feels suffocating, it may well be exposing the burden of the mass or collective consciousness we may carry or over-identify with, which we need to move through to approach ascension.

Chakras that are activated or affected by Rose Essential oil are: **Third Eye Chakra, Throat Chakra, Heart Chakra, Sacral Chakra, Base Chakra,** the **Link Chakra** and the **Earthing Chakras.** The Chakra behind the back of the throat is particularly assisted to throw off the energetic debris of others that may have been inadvertently picked up.

Used on any of the following meridians yields great results physically and energetically: kidney, spleen, liver, lung, bladder, triple warmer and the Governing meridian.

Most of the energy bodies are supported with Rose oil, particularly the etheric field, the causal and spiritual bodies, and most of the light frequencies held within these bodies are increased and enhanced. A higher and finer vibration is also easier to assimilate into the auric fields.

More on Rose Otto Essential Oil

Avicenna (980-1037) the Persian alchemist, astronomer, philosopher, mathematician, physician and poet, who wrote the famous 'Canon of Medicine', used essential oils extensively in his practice. He wrote around a hundred books, with one entirely devoted to roses.

Rose has also been described as 'The Empress' of Essential Oils, because of its wide ranging capabilities. History teaches us of the value placed on the essence and oil of Roses as well as the petals and flowers, with the stories of their use in baths (Cleopatra and her milk baths), romantic settings, perfumes, cooking (Turkish Delight etc) as well as the beauty of the bloom to the naked eye.

There is an increase of Roses around nowadays that do not have any perfume, and though they are certainly beautiful, the specific breeding in this way has compromised the energetic effectiveness on a sensory, auric and olfactory level, placing more emphasis on the visual level.

This has placed more demand on the perfumed roses used for Rose Essential Oils, and rightly so, as they are so amazingly versatile and comprehensive.

Rose Flower Essence

When used as a flower essence it can further assist and enhance most other vibrational remedies being undertaken. This is because it provides support for the **Chakras** and energy centers, together with the protectiveness needed to process gently but surely in the presence of love, grace or acceptance.

Rose Water Therapy

Rose water of good therapeutic, cooking or oral application quality can be used as part of a healing process. If you decide to try using the Rose Water as a detoxification supplement, be aware to take great care and go slowly, as it will dislodge all that is not of love and acceptance within from the physical cells. Even just a few drops in water daily or regularly can begin a huge transformation process. But care must be taken to navigate and monitor the energetic releases or fall-out from this process.

It is wise to work with it energetically and etherically first before using it physically in this way, so that your energy bodies do not get overloaded with trying to process both the physical departing resonances as well as the energetic residues that will be released.

Even just a quarter teaspoon taken daily in water will begin to move stuff out of the physical body at a cellular level quickly, so initially give yourself time to build up to this measure as a regular daily dose, or if you dare to even go beyond the quarter teaspoon measure.

Maybe start off with a few drops in a glass of water every few days initially, and observe the effect first before increasing amount or frequency. Just like the essential oils and flower essences, Rose Water also brings in Divine Love, though it acts directly on the cellular and organ level. This can cause a major detoxification if not handled carefully and wisely.

ROSEMARY ESSENTIAL OIL

Essence of Rosemary Essential Oil

Rosemary has often been associated with the meaning – 'Remembrance'. One of the names origins is claimed to be from the Latin for *'rosemarinus': 'mist of the sea'*. It has been used for honoring and remembering at weddings, funerals and special anniversary ceremonies.

Interestingly it is in some ways connected with memory when it comes to its effects as an essential oil. I would like to offer my interpretation here.

The actions of the oil are simple, yet profound.

Etheric Colours and Properties of Rosemary Essential Oil

Colour Codes; Spring Green, Pearl-Silver, Royal-Blue to Peacock Blue

Starting off with Spring Green, the energy bodies are enlivened and nourished. Placing emphasis upon the heart with this colour code frees it up and this can now allow space for self-love.

From the Green a Pearly-Silver thread arises which funnels out and upward and then fans out into a beautiful mid to Royal Blue with fringed edges of Silver.

As the Green and pearl-Silver is absorbed into the energy fields, the Blue aspects begin to settle into Peacock Blue. This action of the Silvers and Blue tends to leave an imprint (like a fan, or large flat-ish spiral) in the aura for some time. This can last up to 6 hours, depending on the quality and quantity of the oil and its etheric energy that is drawn in through using conscious breathing or intention, or the length of time devoted to working with it.

Pearl colour code brings kindness into the equation, so as it follows on from Spring Green, it allows the kindness to be absorbed into the self through the heart. And lends gentleness in our treatment of the Soul.

Actions & Effects of Rosemary Essential Oil

Action Keywords; *Soul Communication and Healing, Loyalty Discernment & Betrayal, Renewal, Recovery*

The action appears to be working on a Soul level rather than on a Mind or Mental level as more spiritual energy is accessed.

Because of the colour code language and sequencing of Rosemary, nourishing and loving the self can be activated. This results in an etheric energy that is fortifying, allowing for relationship grief to be eased. Working consciously, betrayal and shame through relationships can be tackled, including those that relate to blood ties & incest survival.

Issues of loyalty can be addressed. Loyalty to one's own truth is fortified, bringing in the opportunity for better connection with one's purpose.

Discernment of miss-placed or appropriate loyalty to others are ready to be attended to. The issues and restrictions caused by loyalty incorrectly placed can be reworked, and codependency, betrayal and grief can be dealt with.

Though Rosemary Essential Oil can seem to be about triggering memories, in actuality its effects are in de-stressing and easing painful memories.

When you inhale the etheric energies, the recognition of the first energies of spring Green immediately starts an accessing and clearing process around shock, trauma or other painful memories connected or arising from the memory. This action is different to the action of Clary

Sage or Peppermint, which are both really good for clearing the Mental Body, and helping to settle an overwhelm of thoughts and thought-processing. The action of Rosemary goes to a different level, a level specifically connected to the past.

Right now, with so many light seekers experiencing and dealing with (for a final round) the old **Soul** Memories of past contracts regarding purpose, destiny, oaths and allegiances to past causes etc, Rosemary can assist in settling some of the energetic angst connected with these past memories.

Other related issues that benefit from using Rosemary energetically and consciously are: heartbreak, closure, attachments, self protection, spiritual growth, chocolate, dairy & fat cravings due to the issues covered.

Chakras that are activated or affected by Rosemary Essential oil are: **Earth Star Chakra, Solar Plexus Chakra, Heart Chakra** and some of the **Minor Chakras**.

Meridians: Rosemary also acts on the blood, and supports the spleen, lung, bladder and Governing meridians.

The emotional body and the etheric body are also supported with Rosemary.

More on Rosemary Essential Oil

Soul Communication

Differing essential oil qualities will have varying amounts of Silver within the etheric energies given off. Silver usually denotes flexibility in communication, and this can apply not just outwardly in our external communications, but also inwardly between the various aspects of oneself. This can mean a greater sense of ease within.

Silver is also often connected with balancing the expression of the emotions, the voice of the Soul and with Soul Communication. Used here this denotes a sense of deeper connection and communion with oneself on a Soul level. Happily, too, this also means better soul to soul communication.

In addition, sometimes the dishonesty of another soul may be made clearer through using this oil. But along with this revelation or realization can often appear the means with which to cope with and move through it.

Loyalty to One's Truth and Self Healing / Soul Healing

The main action appears to me to be one of renewal, release, refreshment from past grief, restrictions, betrayals or promises, not only in connection to others, but also to oneself.

When worked with consciously and energetically Rosemary will aid in granting you the space to hear your own Soul Truth again, and assist you to reconnect to your Higher Wisdom.

It is a great essential oil to use as a self healing technique, and perfect for the energy shifts right now!

Cooking Tip:

I have used some of my woodier Rosemary twigs as skewers when cooking – simply strip the 'leaves' off twig branches that have a good length to them, leaving tufts at the top, and sharpen the base of the twig – use as a skewer (after soaking in water if dry) and let the aroma blend into the vegetables or food you are roasting or grilling. You can also save the leaves for roasting veggies, too! Yumm!

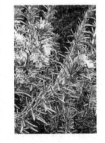

ROSEMARY

SAGE ESSENTIAL OIL

Sage activates the inner wisdom, bringing the Sage of one's being into the light. Ancient knowledge resources are unlocked and used in meditative moments, can assist with ancestral wisdoms and whisperings.

The qualities of sage are well known regarding the cleansing of the aura, and also when used for space clearing. When in concentrated essential oil form, it is focused for deep results within the etheric body.

Etheric Colours of Sage Essential Oil

Colour Codes;   *Yellow Flame, Green, Silver, Electric Spectrum Orange*

The initial colour to reveal itself is the glow of colour of golden Yellow. Like a flame, it surges and twinkles, transforming the mental body. The flame further reaches into the meta-physical realms, allowing clarity and ordering of thoughts, and providing a connection to ancestral information that supports the being.

Green now infuses through the flame and provides space, nurturing and the whisperings of one's inner tuition and direction to break through.

Silver now pulses through, aligning the Soul and its inner wisdoms.

This is followed by Electric Spectrum Orange, which bathes the Sacral area creating a glow around the Tang Tien which empowers the Self again. As all shades of orange reach through the aura, it leaves a glow behind, together with echoes of the Silver afterglow.

Actions & Effects of Sage Essential Oil

Action Keywords;   *DNA Codes, Ancestral Wisdom, Inadequacy, Self Judgment, Denial, Unfocused Direction,*

Self Sabotage, Needs, Expectations Of Others, Legs, Support, Oneness, Resourcefulness

Sage frees the flow of spiritual energy into the physical environment, calms unbalanced psychic energies.

It also releases Psychic contamination and aligns the subtle bodies and strengthens the aura.

Ancient DNA codings of wisdom are activated and align with ancestral knowings for great resourcefulness.

Sage essential oil also acts upon the **Third Eye Chakra**, and behind the head at the **Causal Chakra**. Access to oneness and ancient wisdoms are opened. Sabotages and denials are addressed, self judgment is eased, and one addresses the expectations of others.

The **Zeal Point Chakra** at the back of the body is supported and one is able to access one's own resources.

The **Soul I.D. Point** above the head is affected by the Silver glow, and the personality becomes less hampered by fears or feelings of inadequacy. The **Link Chakra** is also triggered by the combination, bringing balance on multi-dimensional levels which allows for the resources of ancient knowledge to be received via the **Causal** and **Third Eye Chakras**.

More on Sage Essential Oil

Sage cleanses both the aura and the environment.

Digestion is comforted with Sage, allowing better physical and metaphysical assimilation. Change is more easily digested.

Used with a carrier oil as a massage oil, Sage can alleviate back pain when applied to the bladder meridian. It also aids poor circulation in the feet, and can enhance energy flow in the legs when applied to the stomach and bladder meridians.

The conflicts between inner desires and pressures regarding others are eased.

The spine can also benefit from this as a massage oil, promoting better balanced overall energy flow. Do this by holding one hand at the sacrum while the other hand moves the energy upward along the spine to clear any energetic blocks. As the hand reaches the base of the skull, imagine the energy moving up and down the spine between both hands. Gentle rocking of the body whilst working with Sage can also aid in energy blockage releases.

Chakras: **Causal, Third Eye, Zeal Point Chakra, and Soul Point Chakra.**

Meridians: The sciatic nerve also benefits with massage along the gall bladder meridian. Lung and large intestine meridians allow one to 'let go and let flow/come'.

The womb energy in women can be soothed, and any etheric birthing damage can be repaired; massage into Central, spleen and liver meridians, as well as the abdominal region in general.

Precautions:

Do not use during pregnancy, or with children. Avoid direct skin contact without dilution. Avoid in cases of suspected epilepsy. If there is high blood pressure take care if using in the bath, and do not inhale.

Secrets Beyond Aromatherapy

SANDALWOOD ESSENTIAL OIL

Sandalwood has a rich religious tradition, and is also used as a therapeutic application in the Indian Ayurvedic system. It is associated with many cultures and often smells 'familiar' to people.

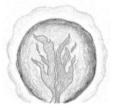

It works with the Kundalini energy and also balances and grounds it.

Sandalwood

Etheric Colours of Sandalwood Essential Oil

Colour Codes; *Orange-Pink, Purple, Green*

The etheric code of Orange brings with it energy for the Sacral Chakra, and with this, it a greater contentment within and with the self. Emerging as it does with a twin plume of Pink, which works on the higher heart; this allows more self love into the moment, as the combination of these colours creates Coral.

The next etheric wave is Purple, which is immediately followed up by Green, in a way that appears to combine them both.

This has the effect of opening the heart space to Divine Source and Oneness whilst transforming and rejuvenating the emotions and our attitude to them, and our physical body and its needs.

Actions & Effects of Sandalwood Essential Oil

Action Keywords; *Divine Sensuality, True Love, Sexuality, Calms Urges, Grounds, Kundalini*

The colour combinations of Sandalwood can help to transmute how we feel within the body, contacting more satisfaction. As it eases our attitudes to relating, it also brings Divine aspects and an almost sacred sensuality and calmness into one's experience of love.

It calms our urges and grounds the Kundalini. This also allows for acceptance of true love, and access to a sense of Divine Sensuality.

Intuition is enhanced as the mental body's control loosens, sensuality becomes more enjoyable and karma is more easily cleared from the Chakras.

The female aspects in the **Sacral Chakra** and the male energies in the **Root (Base) Chakra** are aligned with the **Heart Chakra** and the **Higher Heart space.**

Sandalwood's ability to ground into the **5th Earthing Chakra** helps to aligns us to this planetary anchor chakra that bridges 3D, 4D and 5D aspects of our energy beings.

Meridians that gain most benefit when used in acupressure or massage include: Governing, lung, heart, liver, gall bladder and large intestine.

More on Sandalwood Essential Oil

Meridian work is well supported with Sandalwood. Especially the bladder meridian, small intestine and liver meridians – assisting with frigidity or virility, and also sexual issues and complexes. Applied to the pericardium (heart) meridian, it can assist with intimacy.

This oil acts on all of the Chakras. Performing breathing exercises after applying to the lung reflex points on the hands or feet enhances relaxation.

Yarrow Essential Oil

This delicate and unusual oil is not clear or yellowish like most other essential oils.

Expensive and not easy to track, it is worth the effort and cost for what it returns to those in need.

Its surprise is its delightful rich Blue colour.

I first learned of this oil when researching for the best oils to use for energetic protection many, many years ago.

It is excellent for the LightWorkers and the over-sensitive person and soul.

Etheric Colours of Yarrow Essential Oil

Colour Codes; *Blue-Mauve into Silver with Copper hints, moving into Gold*

Mauve is generally a pinkish variety of Violet, but this Mauve has a Blue -ish iridescence to it.

This etheric code combines the protective and calming effects of blue with the higher vibrations of the Violet-Pink encodings.

Opening up to greater access of various types of Chi, the Silver now emerges to strengthen this action and to align the Soul, anchoring it to the **5th Earthing Chakra** in 3rd and 4th Dimensions.

The Copper hints within the Silver rebuild where overexposure to electrical or electronic interference has weakened.

As the waves move into the Gold frequency, the aura can be healed and sealed when worked with consciously.

Actions & Effects of Yarrow Essential Oil

Action Keywords; *Psychic Protection, Wound Healer, Light Workers, Love & Clairvoyance, Ward Off Negativity, Enhance Clairvoyance, Seeking External Protection, Over-Sensitivity, Aura Compromise From Trauma Or Injury, Seals Energy Breaks In Aura, Overall Energy Fields Strengthener*

Yarrow is good for psychic protection & oversensitivity, as it strengthens the aura & awakens emotional clarity. Great for those who are oversensitive to the environment and are always seeking for protection from outside rather than from within the self, this always protection whilst developing those inner skills.

Yarrow helps us to be our own source of protection. It also wards off negativity and enhances positive perceptions, which helps us to build up our inner resources and core to withstand external pressures more confidently.

As seen by the keywords, it also aids where damage has taken place, rebuilding Auric integrity that has been compromised by injury or trauma in this or another lifetime. Healing and sealing energy breaks, Yarrow strengthens the energy bodies overall.

This essential oil pulls in Heaven Chi, Earth Chi and also Protective Chi. This assists in utilizing Functional Chi as the energy systems work more co-operatively together.

Chakras supported and activated by this oil are: **Crown Chakra, Heart Chakra, Sacral Chakra, Link Chakra** and **5th Earthing Chakra.**

Works directly on the etheric body, mental body, Soul Body and the **new Gridding systems** within the Crystalline Body.

Meridians supported with Yarrow are Central and Governing, lungs, spleen, circulation and liver.

More on Yarrow Essential Oil

Massaged all around the throat and neck, and behind the back of the skull, as well as the feet will assist in aligning and integrating the energy systems quickly.

Applied in carrier oil to the palms of the hands, it can aid in energy work and assist with caring professions by supporting the energy worker or carer and enhancing healing skills.

<><><>

Secrets Beyond Aromatherapy

YLANGYLANG ESSENTIAL OIL

The Nervous System and the emotions are soothed and sedated with YlangYlang. This essential oil is often used in perfumes, and always brings a sense of luxuriousness, sweetness and delight.

Etheric Colours of YlangYlang Essential Oil

Colour Codes; *Gold, Magenta, Green, Purple*

The empowering aspects of Gold immediately stimulates regeneration of the subtle bodies. The entire energy body is bathed and strengthened and more light enters. The Gold infuses through the bodies, leaving residual tinges of golden light in the aura.

As Magenta spirals through the Gold, it builds a bridge to spiritual love, which now impacts on the energy bodies.

Fading into a Green that possesses the vividness of a cut emerald, the heart centre opens to more of love. As this frequency bathes the energy bodies, clear and serene violet-like Purple opens the inner doors. Access to intuition, inner poetry, inspiration, mysticism and transformation is possible.

Actions & Effects of YlangYlang Essential Oil

Action Keywords; *Calm Nerves, Integrate Emotions, Fears, EMF Revitalized, Anger, Frustration, Intimacy, Rejection, Jealousy, Boundaries, Own Destiny*

When the **Nervous System** is calmed in this pleasurable way, the electromagnetic body is revived and recharged. Emotions can then be integrated with less frustration and 'rawness'. And the body and being can begin its renewal again.

The physical body starts to relax, making more of one's healing energy available. The mental body also begins to settle and quieten, releasing concerns whilst providing insights into issues.

YlangYlang calms all of the energy bodies. Less reactivity allows for clearer solutions. Sleep comes more easily.

Feelings of anger, frustration, jealousy and rejection can be viewed differently as one lays aside ones initial stance or reaction, and new choices can be made.

If allowed, it can sublimate the senses, aiding intimacy issues.

Chakras: YlangYlang affects all **Major Chakras**, and some of the new Human chakra anatomy including the **Link Chakra**, which aids in bringing in a better connection to all of one's light bodies. The **Psychic Body Chakras** are cleared and enhanced, aiding psychic possibilities.

Meridians: Used on the following meridians, YlangYlang helps to further support and enhance their better functioning: liver, Governing, pericardium.

More on YlangYlang Essential Oil

Massage around the chest and breast region can remind the body (again) of pleasure, aiding in easing the pain of lost love. Applied all around the hairline, it may assist with unsettling thoughts.

The liver, spleen, gall bladder, Governing and small intestine meridians benefit from YlangYlang, aiding in improving function and releasing emotion overwhelm in the area.

<><><>

Myra Sri

CONCLUSION

In this book you have been introduced to the new evolved Essential Oil Etheric Colours, their Codes of action in certain individual Essential Oils, and the relevant Chakras and Meridian applications wherever possible.

We have looked at several effective methods of application especially for healing and energy work, including specific Energy fields, some of the advanced Evolved Chakras and other impacts that may encompass emotional, neurological, spiritual or even incarnational aspects.

We have examined some ideas relating to the new Era of current incoming energies in the so-named 'New Energy Wave'.

We now have a more advanced picture on how the bountiful and effective Essential Oil can benefit so many aspects of the being on their own personal and spiritual journey.

In these times of talk of 'ascension', it is important to remember that we need to be more fully in our 3D bodies and healing their resistances to be able to house the higher 4D, 5D and certain other frequencies and vibrations.

As many are experiencing the myriad of new symptoms resulting from the conversions of our energy systems to the new and higher 'New Energy Wave' frequencies, it is worth taking note of these new Evolved Chakras too.

This is our new updated etheric technology, dedicated to enabling us to navigate through the energies and shifts of these current vibrational frequencies and resonances – to do so assists us to be better balanced and aligned to these new energies.

It is apparent that we are still in the middle of the influx of these particular frequencies, which are expected to phase out around 2050, allowing the next wave of unique frequencies to become embodied on the planet as well as available for evolving humanity.

Whilst writing I would also like to mention that Crystals have their own story to tell too, as they have experienced their own evolution. You can read about the impacts of the new energies on Crystals in my new book due for publication very soon in 'Crystal Codes – Care, Codes, Ciphers – Aligning to the New Era Energies'.

Thank you, and Blessings as we celebrate the gift of nature's vibrations and their upgraded role in today's quantum healings.

I wish you well on your journey for Light, full health, energy and life.

Good Health,

Myra Sri

GLOSSARY:

Back of the throat (neck):

Refer to the Zeal Chakra Point

Causal Chakra:

The Causal Chakra is situated at the back of the head, in line with the Third Eye Chakra. In most people, it assists with opening to the Higher Self or Divine messages.

Central Chakra Core:

This is the central channel that runs along the spine connecting all of the in-body Major Chakras.

Chakra Core

This is the central channel that runs along the spine connecting all of the in-body Major Chakras.

Ear Chakras:

Part of the Psychic Body Chakra System.

Earthing Chakras:

Part of the New Evolved Chakra System. A requirement to enable correct grounding and anchoring of the Higher Chakras and Main Chakra systems for optimum benefit in the current energy frequencies.

EMF:

EMF is the Electro Magnetic Field – which surrounds all humans and living things. The Human EMF resonates at a different frequency but aims to vibrate in harmony with the Planets. The Earth has her own EMF, and certain oils can assist us to resonate beneficially with the Planet's EMF.

Energetic Action:

Energetic action usually and often includes the meridian systems of the body, the energy flow between the chakras, and any action causing the moving or releasing of energy blockages. Energetic action can occur when a blockage has been stimulated for release. Resulting energy flow movement that affects other energy systems or anatomy further down the line of flow also comes under this action. Etheric action or energetic action on the Etheric level can encompass or affect the Light Bodies as well as the Chakras, and it can also work inter-dimensionally.

Evolved Chakras:

The new evolved Chakras include not only the Higher Chakras, such as the Soul Star, the Cosmic Gateway etc, but also the newly discovered New Earthing Chakras and associated Anatomy, The New Psychic Chakras and Psychic Body Anatomy and The New Signal / Survival Chakras and its associated systems. These are held in a different dimension to the Major Chakras to allow for further spiritual development and evolution as well as providing more comprehensive energy systems to ensure balance during these turbulent and evolving times.

Eye Chakras:

These two Chakras are part of the Psychic Body Chakra System and the Signal Chakra System. These are some of the new evolved Human Chakras in the New Energy Wave.

4 ½ Chakra

Situated around the back of the neck, this is also known as the Psychic Gateway or the Zeal Point. It is related to the Psychic Body and sensory anatomy.

5th Earthing Chakra:

The Fifth Earthing Chakra is a major transducer for our current and Higher Chakra systems. A further book on the new evolved Chakras is being completed for publication soon.

High Heart:

The original 'Heart' Chakra or center was related to the actual physical heart position in the body. The 'High Heart' is the recognized spiritual center which is slightly higher up and more central in position and placement in the body. As we evolve, we have been working with the 'marriage' of the physical heart (our emotional or inner child center) together with the spiritual / higher heart. This alignment is often referred to as the 'Twin Hearts'.

Higher Chakras:

The Higher Chakras are sometimes referred to as the Upper Chakras. These are the energy centres that are outside the body and are situated above the Crown Chakra. They are also sometimes referred to as the 8th Chakra, the 9th Chakra etc and in an evolved or evolving person can number up to the 12th Chakra. Various systems may have different names to them, but these names can include: Soul Star, Even though they are connected to the Crown Chakra they exist on a more refined etheric dimension, which can include 4th and 5th Dimensions.

Link Chakra:

The Link Chakra is a newly discovered Chakra, situated just above and between the knees. Great care must be taken when working with this Chakra as it can be delicate and should not be tampered with by the inexperienced. I will be writing more about this Chakra soon. You can find some information here: http://www.myrasri.com/the-new-vital-chakras

Lunar Energy:

Lunar energy is usually associated or connected with the changing and shifting of emotions, a condition of human life. Using Lunar energy in etheric healing like can assist in going with the flow.

Major Chakra:

The Seven Major Chakras are the currently recognized common or in-body Chakras situated relationally with Nervous System centres.

Minor Chakras:

The minor Chakras usually include Chakras connected with the organs and glands of the body, as well as joints.

Navel Chakra:

The Navel Chakra is not part of the main or normal common Chakra system. Rather it exists on another dimension and connects in with the Soul Body System, the Hara System and the Psychic Body Chakra system. Conception issues as well as early childhood issues may also figure here.

New Evolved Chakras:

These are the new Chakras which have been revealing themselves for the last twenty years or so. There are several systems or bodies of these new energy frequencies, which all inter-relate, though they may perform separate functions. Such energy systems include the new Higher or Upper Chakras – usually Chakras 8th to 12th – the new Earthing Chakras, and other Chakra systems. See Evolved Chakras.

Prana:

Ancient Indian tradition speaks of a universal energy or life-force that is the breath of life. It moves through the body, primarily through the breath.

Self Testing:

A kinesiology tool for self help. A separate book that includes easy Self Testing instructions is also available; *Secrets Behind Energy Fields* by Myra Sri. Alternatively, one can use a Pendulum to test for or verify answers.

Sex Chakra:

The little known Sex Chakra is not to be confused with the Base or Root Chakra, or the Sacral Chakra, this latter being placed approximately between pubic area and navel. Not much has been written about this yet, but will be done so soon. Watch *www.myrasri.com*

Shoulder Chakras:

Part of the Signal Chakra System.

Soul Point Chakra:

This is part of the Soul Body System as well as the Higher/Upper Chakra System. This is also called the Soul I.D. Point, as it is connected with the incarnational identity of the Soul in its current life. It is also sometimes referred to as the Soul Star.

Soul Seat

The Soul Seat is part of the Soul Body anatomy, and sits above the heart and below the throat area. It is a largish area, and we may instinctively put our hands there when we encounter a surprise or shock. Sitting in a different energetic system to the Main Chakra system of the seven Chakras, it can be connected with deep feelings and ancient memories. The Soul Seat and Soul Point Chakras are connected.

Trauma Anchor:

When someone has been forced to do something they didn't want to do, and the body has been held (down, back, tied up, chained etc), it can create an 'anchor' for the emotional memory at the associated points of 'touch' in the physical body. It can register throughout the nervous system and or be more localized in the initial and associated musculature and skin memory.

Such was the case of one small boy who was held by his wrists to be forced to have lots of necessary but very painful injections. His wrists held the traumatic memories as an anchor, and when unwary teachers later went to get hold of him by his wrists, he relived the memory of being held down against his will and responded by becoming quite uncontrollable and wild. Once this was recognized and he was approached in a different way, he ceased this behavior. One would hope that at some time in life he could deal with this memory to allow normal response to touch at these positions.

White-Light:

White-Light contains all of the seven primary colours of the rainbow. These individual colours generally relate to the Seven Major Chakras. This means that each Chakra may receive a minor balance as the White Light passes through a Chakra, or that an individual Chakra will receive a full colour wash which will re-harmonise it again.

Zeal Point Chakra:

The Zeal Point Chakra has also been known as the 4 ½ Chakra or Psychic Gateway Chakra, located at the back of the neck. Some people call this the "widow's hump". It is approximately where the Cervical vertebrae at the neck meets the Thoracic vertebrae or mid to upper spine of the back. This Chakra helps to align the body templates for greater energy flow and assimilation. Outlined in the New Psychic Chakras anatomy and the New Chakras Book. For further developments; http://www.myrasri.com/new-chakras-subtle-body-anatomy

FURTHER INFORMATION

References for this book:

Further posts of information with reference to content in this book:

Ear Chakras: http://www.myrasri.com/extra-ordinary-chakra-balancing

Earthing Chakras: http://www.myrasri.com/new-chakras-subtle-body-anatomy/new-earthing-chakra-system

High Heart Chakra http://www.myrasri.com/extra-ordinary-chakra-balancing

Navel Chakra http://www.myrasri.com/the-new-vital-chakras

New Energy Wave: http://selfhelphealing.net/the-final-energy-waves

Shoulder chakras: http://www.myrasri.com/new-chakras-subtle-body-anatomy/new-signal-chakras-system

COLOUR CHARTS:

You will find the individual artist interpretations (images or illustrations of the etheric colours) of some of the Essential Oils in chart form available for download, together with the Oils Summary Chart in .pdf form at this link:

http://www.myrasri.com/chart-for-book-buyers

<>< ><>

Other Books by the same Author:

Energy Healing Secrets Series

Secrets Behind Energy Fields

Secret Truths – Health and Well-being

New Crystal Codes – Align Your Crystal to the New Era Energies

Secrets to Serene Space – Art of Space Clearing & Creating Sanctuary

Guided Meditations at www.myrasri.com/new-healing-store

Books due for Publication Soon:

The New Evolved Chakras – Chakra Alignment

Affirmations

Want to Know More?

You can sign up for the free newsletter which keeps you informed of periodic special deals and offers, or of the publication of new meditations and books, or other helpful items on life, challenge, change, self help healing, self empowerment and spirituality. You are assured that you will not be harassed, and as your details are treated with confidentiality you are guaranteed that none of your information is shared in any way. You can sign up obligation-free here: www.myrasri.com.

If you would like more information about this or any other book or meditation, please write or email to the author using the following details; admin@myrasri.com

<><><>

About the Author

Myra Sri was born in England and moved to Australia in her twenties with her then husband and two young children. As a sensitive person, she maintained a spiritual leaning.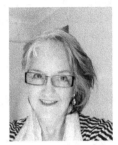

Moving out of her unsupportive marriage and leaving behind her naivety in religious faith she embarked on the reconstruction of her life and the discovery of her true identity.

Continuing to work in the mainstream business, accounting and media industries, she found that connecting with other people further inspired her on her own self development journey and assisting others in their journeys led her to naturally gravitating to the healing professions.

Undertaking extensive training and study she became an energy healing practitioner and kinesiologist. Qualifying as an instructor in several modalities, she subsequently discovered where there was a lack of teaching and understanding and set upon research and discovery, resulting in her own unique advanced workshops which have been taught around Australia since the early 1990's. These continuing experiences led her to develop her own innate skills and supported her in re-membering her healing skills and psychic abilities.

Running her own private practice since the late 80's, Myra remains an avid explorer and student of evolving ways to heal and support the soul and spirit.

She wrote her first book in 2006. Regular trips to the UK concerned family issues until both her parents died and after further teaching and training in England and Germany Myra returned to Australia being freshly inspired to document and write about her new learnings, discoveries and insights, including the current energy shifts since the turn of the millennium affecting essential oils and crystal energies as well as the emergence of the new evolved Chakras.

She embarked on the Energy Healing Secrets Series in 2012 which fulfils part of her role as a Transformation Agent. The Energy Healing Secrets Series is presented to assist in self help, self healing and spiritual mastery.

With the advent of the new era energies and her discovery of the new evolved Chakra systems, she has written and developed the *New Evolved Chakras Workshop series* which includes the new Earthing Chakras, the Psychic Body Chakras and the Signal-Survival Chakras. The discovery of these extraordinary Chakras have also been confirmed by other spiritual teachers and psychics to be instrumental in everybody's healing process and the book on these Chakras is soon to be published.

Myra provides a safe and attentive healing space for her clients and students, and works multi-dimensionally, enabling major energy and spiritual shifts. Her focus is on the Soul and spirit. Considered a knowledgeable and intuitive resource for difficult or complicated situations, she has often been referred to as 'the Healer's Healer'. She works multi-dimensionally, enabling major energy and spiritual shifts.

Workshops

Some of Myra's workshops include:

Past Life Training – Navigating Soul Journey and Genetic Issues and Karma safely

HygienEthics Series (Protection and Energy Management Series) – Working With Energy, Living With Energy, Being Energy, Protection HygienEthics, HygienEthics for Therapists, Advanced HygienEthics

Navigating Life in a Changing World

Muscle Testing Basics

Crystal Workshop

New Evolved Chakra Series - New Earthing Chakras, New Psychic Body and Chakras, New Signal-Survival Chakras

SECRETS BEHIND ENERGY FIELDS

When we have good health, we really do have a huge asset at the ready – there is no price to be placed on it as from our good health so many positive things can arise. When we are exhausted and tired through dealing with other peoples issues, emotions and energies, we are cheating ourselves of our true destiny and life journey.

Nobody lives as an entire isolated and energetic island to themselves. We are all social beings and part of life is social interaction of some kind or another. Which also means energetic interaction - the contact that takes place on those unseen levels, yet we can still feel their action and their impact.

When we don't know where our energy goes, when we work with others closely, when we are faced with emotional or traumatic scenes, when others think it is ok and acceptable to explode around us, when we think there must be something wrong with us because of what we continually encounter in our life, we need answers to what is happening, and what we can do about it!

Learning to navigate through life in energies that are less than positive or harmonious sometimes requires outside information or help. And all you really need to invest is some of your time and energy to become your own energy guru and healer.

Here is a collection of techniques, exercises and tools that are proven energy strengtheners. Selected from the many workshops I have taught on this topic are easy, effective solutions and understandings for anybody who is involved with other people and not coping as well as they could.

You can begin to reclaim your own identity and autonomy again, and easily recognise who and what has been affecting you with the easy to follow instructions and ideas.

Be successful and happy, protect your energy and let good health and good energy be your positive foundation.

If you are doing everything "right" and yet there is something that cannot be explained that compromises your experience of life and vitality, you may well need to look deeper... look past symptoms, past the apparent, past expecting a pill to fix what you can do for yourself.

Exhaustion and tiredness can have several causes. Compromised health can often find us resorting to the local doctor or our health food store. Energetic and emotional impacts, toxicity or damage from others may need to be addressed and resolved separately (*"Secrets behind Energy Fields"*).

We are not just our body, we are not just our mind, we are not just our emotions. We are an amazing combination of all of these and more. The being is an amazing orchestration of matter and that unseen life-force; spirit. When one part is hurt, the other parts are affected.

Here in this book we look at important and often hidden contributors to compromised health and equilibrium as well as very real yet often hidden aspects of tiredness, exhaustion and depletion of energy. Many are not aware of simple things that one can fix for oneself. Nor how easy it can be to make a few mental or verbal changes for oneself that creates a positive impact on health outcomes.

If the nervous system is compromised by amalgam fillings, or lack of hydration, or unresolved issues, then results will be way short of what is possible. If the mind is blocked through lack of simple yet essential nutrients, and is not even aware of essential requirements for health, if a person cannot recognise when they have adrenal exhaustion and how their thoughts can feed into this, what chance does one have of full recovery?

Here is a mix of experiential physical advice and of energetic and spiritual tips from a long-standing expert on body-mind-spirit issues, written to help those who wish to find answers to their problems or symptoms on the *physical level* themselves.

SECRETS TO SERENE SPACE

A new look at the Art of Space Clearing. Clear Negative Energies and Use Metaphysics to Change Your Space and Life.

Become your own Guru. Learn the Art of Creating Sanctuary, within and without...

A home is a place to return to for safety, nurturing, rejuvenation and love. Does your home sanctuary nurture and support you? Does it fill you with pleasure and enjoyment?

Take a moment to look around your home... how does it reflect you? How does it feel to you? Are you able to revitalise and rejuvenate there whenever you need to? Does your home welcome you?

If the answer is "No" and you are aware that you need to do something to change your space, and possibly yourself, then you will find lots of ideas and help in this book.

If you want to go deeper than just shifting surface stuff around, if you feel that there could be some old "nasties" lying around somewhere that you would like to shift, if you feel that you would like to get clearer within yourself as well as within your living space, then this is the book for you!

Decluttering may be needed, or Feng Shui. Or it could be that there are some old or negative energies to clear. What about the sense of being "spied" on? Learn about how to remove not only "nasties" but also learn what a Portal is and how to clear these, as well as Orbs and Thoughtforms.

Discover not only how to Clear your place and enhance your home and life, but the crucial and essential step that must follow for true and lasting success in your Clearing.

Here in an easy to read book you will find how to create Sanctuary in your own personal space. These are time-proven tools, brought to you by an energy expert with many years experience. Decluttering is made easy. Imprints are explained and removal instructions are included together with further powerful techniques to incorporate into your ritual or chosen exercise to bring healing into the home.

This is a true self help book!

NEW CRYSTAL CODES

Since the huge energy shifts of recent years, frequencies have been updated in many areas. The discovery of the new Evolved Chakras has demonstrated that we are all in a process of upgrade and re-alignment. This includes not only the human subtle bodies but also the energetic frequencies of oils and crystals.

This book contains clear instructions on How to Align your Evolved Crystal to the New Incoming Energies.

The author shares her knowledge on the new Crystal Codes and Ciphers, as well as how to read where your crystals energies are at and how to align them with the new Era frequencies.

You will not find this knowledge anywhere else.

This little book also has everything you need to identify the different functions and powers of Quartz Crystals and much, much more.

You will learn about how to connect to your crystal, how to care for it, code and program it and how to use it wisely.

You will find in these pages ideas that will inspire you to love and journey with your chosen gem.

You will also learn how to identify various types of crystals, some metaphysical properties, sets of crystals and learn the difference between an Isis crystal, a Record-Keeper, a Lemurian and much more...

Make the most of your willing crystal and harness its energies for the new energy shifts right now!

This is cutting edge information and the time is ripe to re-energise your crystal.

SECRETS Beyond Aromatherapy

CHAKRA HEALING SECRETS
ETHERIC COLOUR CODES
TRANSFORMATION SECRETS

Behind the Invisible Etheric Codes
of Essential Oils
Chakra and Energy Healing Secrets
for the New Era

MYRA SRI

Secrets Behind Energy Fields

BECOME YOUR OWN ENERGY GURU
RECLAIM YOUR ENERGY & VITALITY

SRI

SECRETS to SERENE SPACE

E CLEARING
VE ENERGIE
SICS AND
O CHANGE
ND LIFE

SECRET Truths Health & Well-Being

HEALTH TRUTHS THAT EVERYONE SHOULD KNOW
TOXICITY AND THE NERVOUS SYSTEM
SECRETS BEYOND NUTRITION

Resolve Exhaustion and Tiredness NATURALLY!
Recognise Obstacles to Health and Vitality
Body-Mind and Emotional Impact

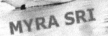

MYRA SRI

The NEW CRYSTAL CODES

Align Your Crystals
To The New Energies

CRYSTAL CODES, CIPHERS AND FUNCTIONS
FOR THE NEW ERA
New: ALIGN YOUR CRYSTALS
CHOOSING AND WORKING WITH CRYSTAL

Learn the difference between an Obi, a Record Keeper, a Tanzanian
and many more.
Sets of crystals to assist in love, success, protection, life stress

MYRA SRI

CPSIA information can be obtained
at www.ICGtesting.com
Printed in the USA
LVHW020010190520
655845LV00006B/233